D0206908

Healing as Vocation

PRACTICING

BIOETHICS

Practicing Bioethics
General Editor: Mark G. Kuczewski, Ph.D.
Neiswanger Institute for Bioethics and Health Policy
Loyola University Chicago

The Practicing Bioethics series provides readers with insight into the professional practices by which bioethicists, physicians, nurses, and other healthcare practitioners address current ethical issues. These works cut through the usual back-and-forth of abstract arguments to examine how to resolve dilemmas in the clinic, at the bedside, and in the boardroom. Volumes address practical issues such as professionalism in healthcare, clinical bioethics consultation, death and dying, and clinical genetics. These books provide a distinctive resource for educating practitioners-in-training such as medical students and residents, allied health professionals, healthcare administrators, and policymakers, as well as students of bioethics at the graduate and undergraduate level.

Editorial Advisory Board

Mark Aulisio, Ph.D., Case Western Reserve University
Rebecca Dresser, J.D., Washington University School of Law
Kevin FitzGerald, S.J., Ph.D., Georgetown University Medical Center
Joel Frader, M.D., Northwestern University, Feinberg School of Medicine
Leslie Francis, J.D., Ph.D., University of Utah
Susan Dorr Goold, M.D., M.H.S.A., M.A., University of Michigan Medical School
D. Micah Hester, Ph.D., University of Arkansas for Medical Sciences
Alex London, Ph.D., Carnegie Mellon University
Laurel Lyckholm, M.D., Virginia Commonwealth University School of Medicine
M. Therese Lysaught, Ph.D., University of Dayton
Kathryn Montgomery, Ph.D., Northwestern University, Feinberg School of Medicine
Daniel Sulmasy, O.F.M., M.D., Ph.D., New York Medical College
Griffin Trotter, M.D., Ph.D., Center for Health Care Ethics, St. Louis University
Delese Wear, Ph.D., Northeastern Ohio Universities College of Medicine
Gladys White, R.N., Ph.D., American Nurses Association

Titles in the Series

Death in the Clinic
 edited by Lynn A. Jansen, 2005
Healing as Vocation: A Medical Professionalism Primer
 edited by Kayhan Parsi and Myles Sheehan, 2006
Living Professionalism: Reflections on the Practice of Medicine
 edited by Patricia M. Surdyk and Erin A. Egan, 2006

Healing as Vocation

A Medical Professionalism Primer

Edited by
Kayhan Parsi and
Myles N. Sheehan

ROWMAN & LITTLEFIELD PUBLISHERS, INC.
Lanham • Boulder • New York • Toronto • Oxford

ROWMAN & LITTLEFIELD PUBLISHERS, INC.

Published in the United States of America
by Rowman & Littlefield Publishers, Inc.
A wholly owned subsidiary of The Rowman & Littlefield Publishing Group, Inc.
4501 Forbes Boulevard, Suite 200, Lanham, Maryland 20706
www.rowmanlittlefield.com

PO Box 317, Oxford
OX2 9RU, UK

Copyright © 2006 by Rowman & Littlefield Publishers, Inc.

All rights reserved. No part of this publication may be reproduced,
stored in a retrieval system, or transmitted in any form or by any
means, electronic, mechanical, photocopying, recording, or otherwise,
without the prior permission of the publisher.

British Library Cataloguing in Publication Information Available

Library of Congress Cataloging-in-Publication Data

Healing as vocation : a medical professionalism primer / edited by Kayan
    Parsi and Myles Sheehan.
      p.   ; cm.—(Practicing bioethics)
    Includes bibliographical references and index.
    ISBN-13: 978-0-7425-3406-3 (cloth : alk. paper)
    ISBN-10: 0-7425-3406-5 (cloth : alk. paper)
    ISBN-13: 978-0-7425-3407-0 (paper : alk. paper)
    ISBN-10: 0-7425-3407-3 (paper : alk. paper)
    1. Physicians—Professional ethics.   2. Medical ethics. I. Parsi, Kayan, 1965–   .
II. Sheehan, Myles N.   III. Series.
[DNLM: 1. Ethics, Medical.   2. Physicians—ethics.   3. Physician's Role.
W 50 H432   2006]
R725.5.H42 2006
610.69—dc22   2006007838

Printed in the United States of America

∞ ™ The paper used in this publication meets the minimum requirements of American
National Standard for Information Sciences—Permanence of Paper for Printed Library
Materials, ANSI/NISO Z39.48-1992.

Contents

Introduction

A recent *New Yorker* cartoon shows a medieval knight mounted on a horse while pounding a hapless serf into submission. Two serfs look on, as one says to the other, "You have to admire his professionalism." Such a tongue-in-cheek appreciation of "professionalism" is rather rare nowadays. Indeed, medical educators are sometimes like the knight in this cartoon—pounding their students into submission with the idea of professionalism without giving them a broader context in which to reflect upon this concept. Rather, professionalism is often presented as pedagogical broccoli to preprofessional and professional students during their training. The typical presentation or article bemoans the denigration of professionalism in medicine because of managed care, the government, or other interests. And despite the avalanche of articles published in the past few years about the topic of professionalism, students often lack a firm grasp of what professionalism in medicine means exactly—historically, sociologically, practically, and personally.

This slim volume (along with its companion volume, *Living Professionalism*, edited by Patricia M. Surdyk and Erin A. Egan) has been prepared to fill this educational gap. Professionalism seems to be on the lips of everyone these days, but perhaps no more so than among medical educators. In preparing this volume as part of a series called "Practicing Bioethics," the editors and authors believe that looking at medicine as a profession dedicated to service and the care of those in need requires descriptive, analytical and reflective approaches. Ideally, emphasizing care and respect for the patient should be enough to lead us to practical decisions about how care should be delivered, patients treated, and relationships between caregivers and those seeking care conducted. Whether this ideal is actually realized by physicians and organized medicine is a question that will be critically examined in this volume.

Perhaps an anecdote would be helpful here. Each year, during our orientation session for new medical students at Loyola University Chicago's Stritch School of Medicine, there is a presentation about medicine and professionalism. Several years ago, one of the students seemed quite annoyed by the presentation. Professions and all this talk about professionalism was, in his view, a ploy by a privileged group to maintain status, secure money and power, and contribute to ongoing structural inequalities in society. There was, he felt, a not so subtle message with which he and members of his class were being indoctrinated that they were better than other people who were not professionals and had more rights and privileges than the rest of the world. The student was, knowingly or unknowingly, echoing an observation of the sociologist Eliot Freidson: "When the leaders of the profession invoke ethics and the values of professionalism, [the] critics declare it is a self-serving ideology that masks the reality of naked self-interest."[1]

The student's comments, and the critique noted by Freidson, point out what could be called the dark side of professionalism. Medical historians remind us that physicians and physician groups have not always risen to the ideals of professionalism in the past. We often act as if only the advent of managed care created challenges to professionalism when, in fact, there have been many such challenges in the past, prior to managed care. As David Rothman notes, where were physicians when there were attempts at universal health care in the 1940s?[2] Or when bad physicians continue to practice? So, this dark side needs to be kept in mind. The purpose of this text is to give the reader the opportunity to explore in depth the idea of medicine as a profession. The editors of this text are fully aware of the failings of the profession of medicine and the misuse of language about professionalism. That is why we present a value-laden introduction for readers that acknowledges the bad uses of professionalism and advocates for a richer and more altruistic perspective.

The presence of this volume, the student's remarks, and the burgeoning literature on the subject of professionalism in medicine indicate that there is a great deal of interest in physicians, medical practice, and the nature of the profession of medicine. That firestorm of interest has been kindled not only because of frustration among physicians and members of the public but also because a feeling exists that we can all do better.

In 1995, addressing the House of Delegates of the American Medical Association (AMA), the late Cardinal Joseph Bernardin spoke about a moral crisis in medicine. His interest in medicine and the profession likely had three sources: 1) concern about another profession, that of the priesthood, and the crisis of abuse that was beginning to shock the Catholic Church; 2) concern about health care, and hospitals in general, arising from his role as archbishop of Chicago and his oversight responsibility for a sprawling collection of hospitals, nursing facilities, and associated social services; and 3) a very personal reason.

In June of 1995, Cardinal Bernardin learned that he had pancreatic cancer and underwent surgery at Loyola University Medical Center. For the next eighteen months, Cardinal Bernardin went through treatment at Loyola, initially chemotherapy and radiation, during which he seemed quite well, and then palliative care after September 1996, when doctors found that a tumor had spread into his liver. Cardinal Bernardin died in December 1996. He was very public about his illness, his experience of health care, and his thoughts about what it was like to be in the hands of the medical profession. His personal experience with the nature of medicine as a profession, along with his own need to reflect on crises in the priesthood and his executive responsibilities for Catholic health care in the greater Chicago area, give a depth and poignancy to his reflections. In his AMA talk, which he delivered when all knew he had pancreatic cancer, Bernardin made it clear that the focus on medicine as a profession was important because "medicine, along with other professions, including my own, is in need of a moral renewal.[3]

Others have picked up on this theme that there is something wrong with the practice of medicine and have raised concerns similar to Bernardin's. One of the contributors to this volume, Matthew Wynia, writing in the *New England Journal of Medicine* some four years after Bernardin's remarks, commented on the growing pressures of profit in medical practice, increasing commercialism, and the lack of health care or coverage for many Americans. Wynia and his coauthors also linked social values with professional values. Medicine's problems in attending to the needy and the poor are a sign of a larger societal problem: "professions protect not only vulnerable persons but also vulnerable social values. . . . When professionalism . . . becomes unsteady, it marks the emergence of societal problems."[4]

Bernardin's and Wynia's comments underscore the fact that at least part of the crisis in the profession has come about because of changes in medical practice over the last ten to twenty years that have made medicine more profit conscious; inspired the growth of for-profit medical corporations with shareholders; and sometimes bewildered individual practitioners and their patients with a proliferation of payment schemes, restrictions on service, growing paperwork, and a confusing network of regulation. The sense of a crisis in medicine is widespread. For physicians, the crisis that some feel is that they are working harder, feel constrained in their ability to care for patients, are controlled and regulated in a variety of ways, and are making less money. For some physicians who truly love what they do, medicine is not fun anymore. For the public, there are concerns about the patient's ability to trust the decisions of the physician, and about whether a physician's recommendation is primarily based on economic considerations or what is best for the patient. And both physicians and patients share concerns, albeit without solutions, as to what seems like a health-care system that is capable of great technological achievements but riddled with issues of quality, access, and, some feel, a lack of human caring.

As previously stated, the problems did not just start a few years ago. Bernardin's and Wynia's remarks focus on the new upsurge of interest in medicine as a profession in the aftermath of a markedly changed business climate and an atmosphere of almost laissez-faire medical capitalism in the United States. This increasingly profit-oriented and business-driven practice of medicine became more prominent in the early 1990s after it became clear that the Clinton administration's proposal for universal health care was going to be soundly defeated.

One should be cautious, however, about overly romanticizing medicine in the past and naively believing that physicians were uniformly altruistic in their practices. What it means to be a physician, how one relates to those for whom one cares, and one's responsibilities to the general public and to other professionals, however, are all items that have been debated in the past. Freidson's critical words about the medical profession suggest that there was no golden age of ideal professionalism in medicine, but a long history of "naked self-interest." However, it does seem to be the case that there is more discontent with and scrutiny of physicians and the profession than there was previously. This scrutiny is due, in part, to lapses in professional behavior that have gone unattended and uncriticized. Medicine has long been viewed by many as a lucrative path to success. There is ample evidence that the profession has not always been very interested in tending to problems of social justice.

In this volume, there will be an opportunity to look more closely at some of the history and roots of medical professionalism, examine some failings, and consider some challenges. In thinking about medicine as a profession, three constructs can be of help: the traditional model, a model based on distinctive moral premises, and a model that looks to the relationship between physician and patient.

A traditional model of medical practice looks to what physicians do individually, how they relate to each other, and the expectations of patients and society for individual practitioners and the profession as a whole. This approach looks to the lived reality of medical practice and can be labeled a sociological model. Four points of this sociological model of the profession stand out. Medicine is seen as a distinctive expertise that requires a long and demanding training. Physicians do things that most people do not have the privilege to do. They take care of the sick, prescribe medication, examine individuals, ask extremely intimate questions, cut people open, and sew them up—these are fairly distinctive traits of physicians. Learning how to do these things safely, competently, efficiently, and with insight as to risks and benefits, requires multiple years of formal education, apprenticeship, and ongoing continuing education.

Second, this type of arduous training provides an expertise that is of great benefit for those who need the services of physicians. Presumably, those who practice medicine prevent disease, limit suffering, prevent premature death, and help the health-care needs of the population.

Third, the kind of expertise that physicians, informed by all the years of acquired knowledge, skills, and attitudes, possess is so complex that both individual physicians and the profession as a whole have considerable autonomy in decision making. Although physicians may currently complain about regulations and limitations on clinical decision making, there still is a remarkable amount of self-determination in following a particular clinical course with a patient.

The fourth characteristic of medicine as a profession is that the autonomy that is given to physicians is part of an informal contract with society. One cannot practice without obligations and responsibilities. Traditionally, those obligations have included caring for those who may put the health of the caregiver at risk (e. g., in an epidemic), providing assistance to the general public health (working to lessen health-care risks, improve sanitation), and rendering assistance in an emergency or to those in desperate straits even if they cannot pay.[5]

Wynia and his colleagues argue for another model of professionalism. This second model emphasizes that in a time of shaky professionalism, one needs to look to moral commitments. Given that the obligations and responsibilities of individual physicians and the profession are currently in danger of being pushed aside by the pressure to make money, either for the physician or for a corporation that controls the physician's services, defining a profession by what it does is not enough. Medicine should not be defined by the distinctive characteristics of its practitioners but by its moral premises.

The contributors of this volume describe, analyze, and reflect upon the profession of medicine and its moral premises in differing but complementary ways. The first chapter, by David Leach, Patricia Surdyk, and Deirdre Lynch, begins with a description of professionalism by the Accreditation Council on Graduate Medical Education (ACGME). The ACGME has played a pivotal role in developing standards for professionalism. The authors focus on four central ideas: 1) Medicine is a cooperative art. Relationships are crucial. 2) Professionalism requires habituation of virtuous behavior. 3) Acquiring professionalism requires regular evaluation and feedback. And 4) caring and competence must come together to create true professionalism. These ideas provide the framework for their discussion in this chapter.

Richard and Sylvia Cruess examine the notion of a social contract between society and the medical profession. They argue that both society and the profession of medicine have certain expectations of each other. Trust plays a pivotal role in this relationship. Without this trust, it is impossible to maintain this fragile social contract. In the following chapter, Matthew Wynia builds upon the idea of a social contract by discussing the formalization of a social contract between medicine and society. He argues that the creation of a national code of medical ethics by the American Medical Association in 1847 was a revolutionary first step by American physicians to formalize the social contract that the Cruesses discuss. He also examines in some detail the influence of various sociological thinkers upon the idea of professionalism and professions. He argues that despite the decline of membership in professional associations such as the AMA, they serve a useful purpose in contrast to alternative modes of health-care delivery through the market or state.

In his chapter, Frederic Hafferty critically examines the threat of commercialism upon contemporary medicine. He focuses his critical eye on six contemporary professional statements of medicine and considers how commercialism and its threats to medical professionalism are defined and addressed. These six statements are 1) the AMA *Principles of Medical Ethics*, (revised in 2001), 2) the AMA *Declaration of Professional Responsibility: Medicine's Social Contract with Humanity*, 3) the AMA *Code of Medical Ethics: Current Opinions with Annotations (2004 edition)*, 4) the American College of Physicians' *Ethics Manual (Fourth edition)*, 5) the Federation of State Medical Boards' *Guide to the Essentials of Modern Medical Practice (Tenth edition)*, and, finally, 6) the *Medical Professionalism in the New Millennium: A Physician Charter*, created as a collaborative effort by the members of the American Board of Internal Medicine Federation, the American College of Physicians–American Society of Internal Medicine, and the European Federation of Internal Medicine.

Jing-Bao Nie's chapter provides the medical student or resident a rather rare opportunity to learn more about the role that sincerity and authenticity play in traditional Chinese medicine. Nie draws upon the intellectual influence of Sun Simiao, a physician who was born in the sixth century and lived to be over one hundred years old. In addition to being an important clinician, Sun wrote extensively about moral matters in medicine. He stressed sincerity in spirit when dealing with medical matters, whether in developing medical skills during training or when facing potentially dangerous situations. Nie also draws upon the profound influence the major religious traditions of Daoism, Confucianism, and Buddhism have had upon Chinese culture, and their particular emphasis upon sincerity.

The chapters by Mark Kuczewski and Eugene Boisaubin and their respective coauthors offer the reader two different approaches to integrating professionalism in undergraduate and graduate medical education. Kuczewski is the director of the Neiswanger Institute for Bioethics and Health Policy at the Loyola University Chicago Stritch School of Medicine. Stritch is one of a handful of Catholic medical schools in the United States. Boisaubin is an internist and ethicist at the University of Texas Health Science Center in Houston (UTHSC-Houston), a large secular medical school. Kuczewski and his coauthors describe how justice is taught at Stritch by "doing, reflecting, and contextualizing." Students are given opportunities to engage with various activities oriented toward justice and then are asked to reflect and contextualize their experiences. The chapter contains excerpts from students' reflective commentaries about their experiences. The commentaries are powerful and sometimes poignant examples of how students try to make sense of their feelings with regard to justice and health care. Boisaubin and his coauthors describe in detail the implementation of an extensive ethics and professionalism curriculum for students at UTHSC-Houston. They also recount how residents are evaluated by a variety of methods, whether by oneself, one's peers, medical students, or patients. This "360 degree" method provides a broad and varied way to effectively evaluate professionalism among residents.

Lastly, Dewitt Baldwin discusses what he describes as the two faces of professionalism: macroprofessionalism and microprofessionalism. Macroprofessionalism refers to those more public expressions of professionalism, "the standards, the rules, and the roles that social organizations and institutions play in human interactions," as Baldwin puts it. This face of professionalism focuses on the issues that the Cruesses and Wynia raise earlier in the book: What is the meaning of the social contract between society and the professions? What role do professional associations play? Microprofessionalism, on the other hand, deals with the kinds of behaviors and attitudes that physicians display (or do not display) on a daily basis in their clinical work: honesty, integrity, responsibility, trustworthiness, compassion, and cooperation. He relates that much of the professionalism literature focuses on the negative aspects of professionalism rather than the positive. Hopefully, these readings will allow the reader—whether a premed, medical student, resident, practicing physician, or medical educator—to reflect upon how to achieve a more positive and robust sense of professionalism.

I would like to acknowledge our medical students at Loyola University Chicago Stritch School of Medicine for their example and enthusiasm in teaching me about professionalism, the contributors to this volume for their thoughtful work, and Mark Kuczewski for suggesting this volume as part of the Practicing Bioethics series. (MNS)

I would like to thank the editorial staff at Rowman and Littlefield for their help in making this a better book, specifically Kat Macdonald, Emily Ross, and Eve DeVaro. Thanks to Robbin Hiller for her help in carefully proofreading our index. Lastly, I would like to thank my wife Lara Bonasera, MD. Caring for our two young sons while being a compassionate, conscientious, and competent physician is a daily reminder to me of medical professionalism at its finest. (KP)

NOTES

1. E. Freidson, *Professionalism Reborn: Theory, Prophecy, and Policy* (Chicago: University of Chicago Press, 1994). Quoted in M. K. Wynia, S. R. Latham, A. C. Kao, et al., "Medical Professionalism in Society," *New England Journal of Medicine* 341 (1999): 1612–16.

2. D. Rothman, "Medical Professionalism: Focusing on the Real Issues," *New England Journal of Medicine* 342 (2000): 1284–86.

3. J. Bernardin, *Renewing the Covenant with Patients and Society* (St. Louis: Catholic Health Association, 1995).

4. Wynia, Latham, Kao, et al., *Medical professionalism.*

5. D. Ozar and D. Sokol, *Dental Ethics at Chairside: Professional Principles and Practical Applications*, 2nd ed. (Baltimore: Johns Hopkins University Press, 2002).

1

Practicing Professionalism

David C. Leach, Patricia M. Surdyk, and Deirdre C. Lynch

Professionalism expresses itself in action. Medical students and residents grow as professionals by committing acts of professionalism—acts of integrity, respect, compassion, responsiveness, commitment, and excellence—in order to practice and acquire the habit of professionalism. While both medical school and graduate medical education (GME) curricula include content related to professionalism, students and residents can never say they have fully "covered" professionalism as a discrete item in the curriculum; instead, the habit of professionalism constantly emerges, or should emerge, in their daily encounters with patients, colleagues, and teachers. The nature of this competency requires that medical students and residents must engage in regular and disciplined personal reflections and clarifying conversations about their daily experiences in order to develop the habit of professionalism. They must commit to this discipline for life as they constantly strive to become better doctors.

WHAT IS PROFESSIONALISM?

The Accreditation Council for Graduate Medical Education (ACGME) considers professionalism as central to medicine and identifies it as one of six general competencies used to ascertain whether the residency programs it accredits have achieved acceptable educational outcomes. The ACGME's view of professionalism encompasses respect, compassion, integrity, responsiveness, commitment, and excellence (table 1.1).[1] These important and inspiring words, however, lack concrete details to guide the actions of faculty and program directors responsible for the formation of medical students and residents as well as for the students and residents who aspire to achieve such ideals. Where does one look for the details by which to start this lifelong journey or to guide others along the path?

FRAMING THE ISSUE

To become fully professional defines a course of serious work, the most serious work that students and residents will undertake in their careers. Such work requires that one becomes fully human. A little philosophy helps us recognize that this statement is far from an empty cliché. Students and residents come to medicine with three human faculties that constitute the building blocks of professionalism, namely, the intellect, the will, and the imagination. The intellect has as its object, truth; the will, goodness; and the imagination, beauty. Translated: physicians must train their intellect to discern the truth, their will to make good clinical judgments, and their imagination to determine that the daily work of medicine is accomplished with harmony, creativity, and beauty. These three attributes eventually emerge as the sustaining professional values of integrity (discerning and telling the truth), altruism (putting what is good for the patient before what is good for the doctor), and practical wisdom, or prudence (beauty in clinical judgment). Professionalism is about the behavior, values, and rules that help integrate all these faculties into what Aristotle (whose father was a physician) would call *arête,* or true excellence.[2]

Medical students and residents can be thought of as amateurs entering a

Table 1.1.   ACGME Description of Professionalism

Residents must demonstrate a commitment to carrying out professional responsibilities, adherence to ethical principles, and sensitivity to a diverse patient population. Residents are expected to:

Demonstrate respect, compassion, and integrity; a responsiveness to the needs of patients and society that supersedes self-interest; accountability to patients, society, and the profession; and a commitment to excellence and on-going professional development.

Demonstrate a commitment to ethical principles pertaining to provision or withholding of clinical care, confidentiality of patient information, informed consent, and business practices

Demonstrate sensitivity and responsiveness to patients' culture, age, gender, and disabilities.

formative process that results in developing the habit of professionalism once their humanistic values are expressed, tested, and refined in the complex situations integral to patient care. Professional development is, therefore, dependent on increasingly challenging medical situations that test individual humanistic values. A few general observations might prove particularly helpful in developing the habit of professionalism.

HELPFUL OBSERVATIONS
ABOUT PROFESSIONALISM

Medicine is a cooperative art; becoming professional means paying attention to relationships.

Medicine is a science as well as a cooperative and integrative art. For millennia, its goodness and benefits have depended on collaborative relationships with patients, colleagues, and others. Medicine cooperates with and enhances the body's natural tendency to heal. Clinical outcomes are not solely dependent on the doctor; they are the "product" of relationships. The quality of patient care depends on the quality of the relationships supporting that care; professionalism is all about relationships.

Kuczewski frames professionalism as "the norms of the relationships in which physicians engage in the care of patients."[3] We have expanded this framework to suggest that professionalism is also evident in a physician's relationships with other health-care providers, with colleagues, students and teachers, with him- or herself, and with society.[4] These interdependent relationships form the context of professionalism and influence its development.

As the body has a natural tendency to heal, so too most students and residents have a natural tendency to ascend to integrity, altruism, and practical wisdom, to move toward *arête*. If the patterns of relationships in a given institution are unprofessional, for whatever reason, the student or resident will find it much harder to practice professionalism than if the institution takes professionalism seriously by expecting and supporting it. For instance, the relationships of medicine are increasingly housed in corporate organizational models. The corporate model tends to emphasize competitive production over compassionate cooperation. This shift presents a unique contemporary challenge to medical professionalism. If the student or resident lacks the tendencies toward *arête*, or if the teachers, staff, and environment fail to support that ascension, professional development will be thwarted.

One way to monitor the quality of the relationships in the community is to monitor the quality of the daily conversations—conversations with patients, with colleagues, and with teachers. Do conversations clarify integrity, altruism, and practical wisdom? Good communities clarify experience; good communities foster professionalism.

Professionalism is a habit; competence in professionalism might mean changing habits, not simply acquiring knowledge and skill.

To make progress in the competency of professionalism, students and residents need to pay attention to their habits. By the time they enter medical school, students have acquired habits that affect their relationships with peers, nurses, other health professionals, and with patients. During residency they further develop these habits or acquire others, based often on what they observe in their work environment or whom they choose to emulate. These habits, while modifiable, reveal patterns of relating, especially under the stress of clinical work, patterns that reflect values such as respect, compassion, commitment, integrity, and excellence. Habits are related to character; professionalism can be thought of as character development occurring in the context of the work of patient care.

The habit of professionalism will emerge only by spending time and energy reflecting on clinical experiences, both individually and in the community, only by consciously fostering integrity, altruism, and practical wisdom, and only by consciously becoming fully human, uniquely and fully available to patients and colleagues.

Acquiring competence in professionalism requires regular assessment of behaviors; evaluations by oneself and others shape performance.

Performance of each of the competencies of medicine is enhanced by feedback, which is essential for professionalism. Because professional behaviors emerge in the context of relationships, it is necessary to assess their development in relationships. The process must begin where it starts, with oneself and with self-assessment. Some students have found it helpful to spend a few moments at the end of each day asking two questions: What things did I do well today? What can I improve? Doing this for each of the domains of integrity, altruism, practical wisdom, and attention to relationships is formative. Keeping a journal enables students to notice patterns over time.

Regular conversations with others help. Another student, a resident, a faculty member—all can help clarify experiences to deepen one's understanding of professionalism. Sharing one's perceptions with others helps to clarify them. Students and residents who seek input from others have the benefit of receiving their perceptions about both the general situation and their particular behaviors therein; 360-degree confidential evaluations from nurses, peers, supervisors, and patients broaden the scope of feedback obtained and provide students and residents with useful data for the work of formation.[5] A portfolio of cases that illustrates issues in professionalism can be useful. Narrative reflections on challenges faced, their resolution, and characteristics of the system that helped or inhibited professionalism are all valuable information that provides reflective material for oneself and useful examples for others in the learning environment. Chisholm and Croskerry offer an instructive example of a portfolio entry that demonstrates reflection, practice analysis, and personal learning points generated from a difficult patient encounter.[6]

Formal evaluation sessions in which students and residents are observed interviewing, examining, or giving advice to a patient or his or her family help document the performance behaviors associated with the habit of professionalism. Standardized patients, simulated conversations, and role-playing present the student and resident with various challenging situations and options in a safe, controlled environment and often reveal the consequences of various options when responding to patients or colleagues and foster reflection on what may be correct or wrong about the various options.

Professionalism occurs when caring meets competence; either alone is insufficient.

Caring for the patient provides an unequaled opportunity for the student or resident and, indeed, is a prerequisite for the formation of professionalism; the act of caring for patients itself, however, is not enough. Patients, peers, the health-care system, and society expect physicians to practice medicine competently; the expectation of competence is the reason why physicians are trusted with what are often the most private and vulnerable moments of a person's life. "Professionalism is the ability to meet [all] the relationship-centered expectations required to practice medicine competently."[7]

What does competence look like? The ACGME and the American Board of Medical Specialties (ABMS, the umbrella organization for certifying boards) agree that competent physicians have abilities in the following areas: medical knowledge, patient care, professionalism, practice-based learning and improvement, interpersonal and communication skills, and systems-based practice. Professionalism integrates all these competencies. It can be observed, for instance, with practice-based learning and improvement when students or residents reflect on their performance and ask themselves, "how could I have done it better?" This requires learners to be honest with themselves, to tell the truth even when they feel inadequate to the tasks at hand.

Professionalism interfaces with systems-based practice when students or residents help patients obtain the care and resources they need to maintain health. Professionalism overlaps with interpersonal and communication skills and with patient care when students or residents are respectful in their interactions with others.

Current standards or expectations for medical knowledge (and in some cases patient care) come from the certifying boards who administer certification examinations. Standards for all the competencies are eminent. The paradox of professionalism is that it demands both standardization and uniqueness. On one hand, physicians are expected to meet standards and adhere to a set of rules and principles that characterize professional behavior. Yet becoming fully professional means becoming more authentically and more uniquely oneself—offering one's unique and authentic response to the challenge of being professional. As Parker Palmer says, being professional involves the skills of the head and hands, yes, but also the skills of the heart.[8]

LEARNING BY EXAMPLE

We often hear it said that values are caught, not taught. Whereas issues of professionalism and related professional content can be taught directly, professional values and behaviors are often learned by example. Medical history is full of such examples, both good and bad. Ignaz Semmelweis (1818–1865) recognized how routine hand washing could significantly decrease infant mortality rates caused by puerperal fever. Despite documented proof from his own clinic, he was denied an academic promotion and was no longer allowed to teach, because his superiors felt that hand washing was not important.[9] Semmelweis went from place to place advocating hand washing, but few listened. He died in an insane asylum at age forty-seven. His commitment to tell the truth and to help patients may not have been related to his ultimate insanity, yet it was clearly related to his failure at academic promotion. Fortunately, such extreme sacrifice is not common, but Semmelweis's story demonstrates the clarifying power of values that inform professionalism.

But it is not necessary to scour medical history to find examples of professionalism. Every year, hundreds of medical students and residents participate in meaningful service projects in their communities. These same individuals become the physicians who continue to donate thousands of pro bono hours in free clinics, in overseas projects, and in fostering improved community health through any number of initiatives. Large academic medical centers, community hospitals, and individual residency programs have curtailed the practice of "drug company lunches" in recognition of research showing that these events, an accepted part of the medical education culture for so long, exercise a subtle but real influence on physicians' prescribing patterns. The examples are often unsung, and they are endless.

The humanistic values upon which professionalism is based are not fragile; they are deeply integrated into human faculties. Yet some suggest that in the process of medical education, these values are often replaced by cynicism. A truer statement might be that most students enter medical school with basic humanistic values, which may or may not survive intact but, in any case, should not be confused with professional values. Developing the habits of professionalism requires that students and residents find support to safeguard their humanistic values. It may take courage, like that demonstrated by Semmelweis, however, to express these values. Unprofessional behaviors are much easier to overlook than to question openly, especially for students or residents who are simply trying to do well in a particular clerkship or on a required rotation. It takes courage to name and inquire into unprofessional behaviors by others, and even more to name one's own inevitable failings. Ongoing conversations with exemplars help develop both clarity and courage—students and residents should find mentors with whom they can reflect on their personal observations and reactions.

On a practical note—students and residents find it useful to let people who want to help them know of their interest in professionalism. Doctors who have mastered professionalism usually stand out and are highly respected by their colleagues. They should be noticed and imitated. We learn by imitating.

CONCLUSION

Medicine is a cooperative art and a deeply satisfying profession. Students become professional by paying attention to the relationships of medicine—relationships with patients, colleagues, and mentors. Competence in professionalism is a habit, and its acquisition requires more than knowledge and skill. Regular assessments by oneself and others are essential. Professionalism integrates all the competencies of medicine and enables one to become the complete physician; indeed, it both enables and requires that the students and residents become fully human.

NOTES

1. The six general competencies, their definitions, references, and assessment tools may be found at www.acgme.org.

2. Aristotle, *The Nicomachean Ethics*, trans. David Ross (Oxford: Oxford University Press, 1998).

3. M. Kuczewski, "Developing Competency in Professionalism: The Promise and the Pitfalls," *ACGME Bulletin,* October 3, 2001; M. Kuczewski, E. Bading, M. Langbein, and B. Henry, "Fostering Professionalism: The Loyola model," *Cambridge Quarterly of Healthcare Ethics* 12 (2) (2003): 161–66.

4. P. M. Surdyk, D. C. Lynch, and D. C. Leach, "Professionalism: Identifying Current Themes," *Current Opinion in Anaesthesiology* 16 (2003): 597–602.

5. D. W. Musick, S. M. McDowell, N. Clark, et al., "Pilot Study of a 360-Degree Assessment Instrument for Physical Medicine and Rehabilitation Residency Programs," *American Journal of Physical Medicine and Rehabilitation* 82 (2003): 394–402.

6. C. D. Chisholm and P. Croskerry, "A Case Study in Medical Error: The Use of the Portfolio Entry," *Academic Emergency Medicine* 11 (2004): 388–92.

7. D. C. Lynch, P. M. Surdyk, and A. Eiser, "Assessing Professionalism: A Review of the Literature," *Medical Teacher* 26 (4) (2004): 366–71.

8. P. J. Palmer, "Reflections on a Program for the Formation of Teachers" (occasional paper, Fetzer Institute, 1992); P. J. Palmer, *A Hidden Wholeness: The Journey Toward an Undivided Life* (San Francisco: Jossey-Bass, 2004).

9. M. Best and D. Neuhauser, "Ignaz Semmelweis and the Birth of Infection Control," *Quality and Safety in Health Care* 13 (June 2004): 233–34.

2

Professionalism and the Social Contract

Sylvia R. Cruess and Richard L. Cruess

THE CONCEPT OF THE SOCIAL CONTRACT

The concept of a social contract was developed by Hobbes, Locke, and Rousseau over three hundred years ago. It attempted to explain the relationship between citizens and those governing them and proposed that this relationship was based on a reciprocal set of rights and privileges.[1] While the concept has lost favor in the realm of political science, it has been resurrected and utilized by social scientists, medical administrators, and physicians to describe the relationship between the medical profession and the society that grants medicine its privileges.[2]

Because of the complexity of its knowledge bases, society has used the concept of the profession as a means of organizing the delivery of selected necessary services, such as law, the ministry, and medicine.[3] When the modern profession was established in the mid-nineteenth century, society granted physicians a monopoly over the use of medicine's knowledge base, autonomy in practice, status, considerable financial rewards, and the privilege of self-regulation on the understanding that the profession would assure the competence of its members, who would be devoted to altruistic service, demonstrate morality and integrity in all their activities, and address issues of societal concern within their domain. This was and has remained the essence of the social contract, which is clearly based on professionalism. Fundamental to this con-

9

cept is trust; society must have trust in individual physicians,[4] and physicians must trust that society will meet their reasonable expectations.[5]

It was not thought necessary to invoke the concept of the social contract until recently. Indeed, professionalism was rarely taught as a specific skill in medical schools or during postgraduate training, although it was frequently invoked, without definition or description, as an ideal to be pursued. Medicine in most countries was a fairly homogenous profession serving societies that themselves were not very diverse. Professionalism and professional values were shared and passed on during the process of socialization by respected role models. Trust in both individual physicians and in the medical profession in the latter part of the nineteenth and most of the twentieth century was high.[6] Clearly the general public believed that the medical profession was not abusing its monopoly and was self-regulating well enough so that standards were acceptable, and that the concept of the profession was worth supporting as a means of organizing the delivery of health care. Difficulties arose throughout the world during the 1960s and 1970s, when an increasingly diverse and "questioning society" greeted traditional values and all sources of authority with skepticism. Because of the status of the professions and the power that they were able to exert, their performance was scrutinized very carefully. Medicine's failures—and they were and are real—were recorded extensively, largely in the social sciences literature.[7] The most telling criticisms were that both individual physicians and the profession as a whole were exploiting their privileged position by pursuing their own self-interests rather than serving the needs of their patients and society; that medicine, having weak standards often capriciously applied, had failed to self-regulate; and that many of medicine's institutions were more devoted to serving their own members than society. Essentially, medicine was accused of failing to fulfill some of its central obligations under the social contract. It was Paul Starr who used the word "contract" for the first time in relation to health care.[8] He stated that the contract was in the process of being revised to better cope with the tensions between the medical profession and society in an increasingly complex and expensive health-care system. Thus the social contract, which has in fact existed since the modern professions were developed in the nineteenth century, was only articulated when the need for change became apparent.

The concept of the social contract has been described as follows: "the rights and duties of the state and its citizens . . . are reciprocal and the recognition of this reciprocity constitutes a relationship which by analogy can be called a social contract."[9] It is difficult to address for two reasons. In the first place, much of it is unwritten and what is in print is found in a wide variety of places—in codes of ethics, legislation granting licensure, the laws establishing the structure of the health-care system, the rules and regulations of Medicare and Medicaid, and a host of other locations. Secondly, the modern contract is constantly evolving as the health-care system changes, as societal needs and expectations alter, and as physicians' expectations change. In spite of these difficulties and differences in cultures and the structure of health-care systems, there are some universal values that remain relatively constant.[10] These values, which medicine and society share, give rise to a set of mutual expectations that, although not always articulated or made explicit, provide the terms of the social contract under which medicine and other professions exist within a society.

SOCIETAL EXPECTATIONS OF MEDICINE

The Services of the Healer

Every physician during his or her practice simultaneously fills two roles—that of the healer and of the professional.[11] The role of the healer has been with us since before recorded history. Western medicine traces its origins to Hellenic Greece, and the Hippocratic and Aesklepian traditions form an important part of medicine's self-image. The professions have different origins, having arisen in the guilds and universities of medieval Europe and England, but had little impact on society, serving only a small elite. As the industrial revolution provided sufficient wealth so that the population at large could purchase health care, science made health care worth purchasing. Society then needed some means of organizing the delivery of these increasingly complex services and turned to the preexisting concept of the profession to accomplish this. At this point, the healer acquired the rights and privileges as well as the obligations of the professional. However, it cannot be stated too strongly that what individual patients want and require is the traditional role of a competent and caring healer. Professionalism is a means to an end.

Assured Competence

Society, acting through the state, has granted the professions the privilege of self-regulation by delegating some of its power to them. As a result, under the social contract, medicine is expected to assure the competence of each practicing physician. It does this by setting and maintaining standards for education, training, and practice. This includes identifying incompetent, unprofessional, or unethical practitioners and either assisting them to correct their deficiencies, or removing them from practice so that they will do no harm.

Each physician must assume individual responsibility to be competent, but society expects more. Practitioners are also responsible for the performance of their colleagues and must both support the profession's self-regulatory activities and participate in them.[12]

Altruistic Service

Physicians are required in the course of the practice of medicine to ask intrusive questions that invade a patient's privacy and to carry out procedures that are invasive in nature. This can only be permitted in an atmosphere of trust, and this trust depends on the patient's belief that the physician will constantly place the patient's interest before his or her own. This is the meaning of altruism. Until a few decades ago, individual physicians demonstrated their altruism by caring for the indigent at no charge. The introduction of Medicare and Medicaid, as well as national health insurance in many countries, has largely removed this opportunity in the developed world. This occurred as medicine was being transformed from a cottage industry to an activity that consumes a significant portion of the wealth of each nation. Physician remuneration increased, both in absolute and relative terms, leading many to feel that the medical profession was abusing its privileged status and monopoly for its own gain at the expense of the public good.

There has always been a conflict between altruism and self-interest, and the recent generation of physicians, feeling that it has the potential to lead to an unhealthy lifestyle, has objected to the open-ended nature of medicine's commitment.[13] As this aspect of the social contract is renegotiated to be more acceptable to younger individuals, it is essential that the public continue to believe that their physicians will be there when they require care. This is central to patient trust and the ability of the physician to heal. Assuring the public of medicine's altruism should be possible, as the public does not put unreasonable demands on physicians, and with proper communication and organization (i.e., group practices, etc.), the public's expectations can be met. Since the assumption of altruism is such an important societal expectation, it becomes incumbent upon each physician to be conscious of its importance in his or her day-to-day life.[14]

The profession as a whole is also expected to demonstrate altruism in its activities. Medicine's institutions and associations must place the welfare of society above that of the profession and its members. There is some evidence that the loss of trust in medicine as a whole during the past few decades resulted not as much from the actions of individual physicians, but from those of medicine's associations, which are believed to have given priority to representing their members rather than societal good, thus breaching the terms of the social contract.[15]

It seems axiomatic that associations are collections of individuals, and consequently, individual physicians must take some responsibility for the performance of their associations.

Morality and Integrity

To support patient trust, the nature of medical work requires that physicians be regarded as demonstrating morality and integrity. This must occur not merely when they are functioning as professionals but in their day-to-day lives as well. It is not possible to maintain trust in a physician whose behavior outside of medicine does not reflect these qualities. As Justice Louis Brandeis believed, professionals are held to higher standards than are members of other occupations, and this represents a major expectation of the public.[16]

Promotion of the Public Good

Under the social contract, licensing laws grant physicians a monopoly over the use of medicine's knowledge base on the clear understanding that this knowledge will be used to address issues promoting the health of individual patients and of society as a whole. Members of the medical profession are thus expected to react to concerns about the structure and cost of the healthcare system, and the state of the nation's health as well as new situations in medicine's domain, such as unexpected epidemics or bioterrorism. In recent years, medicine's advice has frequently been unsolicited or ignored, but individual citizens still expect medicine to use its expertise in an objective fashion for the betterment of society.[17]

In the twenty-first century, when the cost of medical care has imposed limits on the resources available for care, physicians are often faced with a conflict between the needs of an individual patient and the need for society to limit resources.[18] This dilemma will grow in the upcoming decades and will require decisions acceptable to both medicine and society.

Transparency

As self-regulating organizations, the professions traditionally carried out their deliberations in a relatively closed fashion.[19] It seems probable that this was unintentional, as initially there was very little public interest in their activities. However, as increasing levels of accountability were demanded, the medical profession came to be regarded as overly secretive in its processes and as being relatively insensitive to the needs of the public.[20] Criticism was leveled at the methods of setting standards and over disciplinary procedures in many jurisdictions. As a result, public membership on regulatory bodies was either established or increased, and public input into discipline and the setting and maintenance of standards has expanded. As a result of medicine's own initiatives, public pressure, and changes in legislation, the deliberations of most important medical organizations that have an impact on the public are now carried out in a much more open and transparent fashion. This is clearly an important public expectation under the social contract, and it can be anticipated that further changes will occur in the future.

Accountability

The professions have always been accountable to those served. Thus, physicians have answered to their patients, but accountability in contemporary terms has been greatly expanded.[21] Part of this results from the cost of modern health care; part from the information age, which has both informed and empowered patients; and part because of the questioning of all forms of authority that were previously the beneficiaries of 'blind trust.'

Medicine's traditional accountability is to patients and to colleagues for the advice given on public policy and for the results of self-regulatory activities. The well-documented failure to adequately monitor standards of practice, and the abuse of the collegiality inherent in professionalism to protect incompetent, unethical, or unprofessional conduct in highly publicized cases, has lead to an erosion of trust[22] and diminished medicine's ability to influence the newer levels of accountability that have been expected in recent decades.

In addition to the traditional areas, physicians are now accountable in both economic and political terms.[23] The economic accountability is to the current payers for health care—the state and/or the market. Physicians are asked to ensure that their services are cost effective and, to an increasing degree, to include as factors in their decision making the impact of their decisions on the overall economics of health care. In political terms, they have been given responsibility for the health of populations and for some aspects of the overall functioning of the health-care system. Without question, the newer levels of accountability are now regarded as an important aspect of the social contract.[24]

MEDICINE'S EXPECTATIONS UNDER THE SOCIAL CONTRACT

If the concept of a social contract is valid, and if it serves as the basis for societal expectations from individual physicians and the medical profession, it follows that individual physicians and medicine as a profession can also have reasonable expectations from society. There are two points that are worthy of emphasis. In the first place, society's trust in individual physicians and in the profession is heavily influenced by how medicine is perceived to meet its obligations under the contract. It has been observed that medicine's failings have resulted in a loss of trust and that, as a result, the social contract has been altered. However, if physicians are to be expected to put the welfare of others above their own, they themselves must trust the system within which they are working. There is some evidence to indicate that the sense of disillusionment felt by many physicians is due to their belief that society is not meeting some of its obligations.[25] Secondly, if an implicit contract exists, then negotiating the details of this contract becomes a legitimate professional activity.[26] Obviously, the medical profession would be wise to emphasize the nonfinancial aspects of the contract, but ensuring proper conditions of work as well as remuneration is an entirely appropriate activity.[27] However, during these negotiations, which take place in a variety of settings and situations, medicine must place the public interest first, as any other approach is inconsistent with the tradition of the professional.

A Health-Care System That Is Value Driven and Provides Adequate Resources

It is society's right to determine the structure and organization of the health-care system that they desire, and physicians have an obligation to work within the system which is in place.

The entry of the state and the corporate sector into the health-care field has dramatically altered the social contract.[28] Their efforts at cost control using accounting logic[29] have transformed the negotiating table and resulted in a dramatic diminution of medicine's influence in health care. The negotiating stance of the profession has often been regarded as self-serving.

However, the health-care system can subvert the values of the healer and the professional. The drive to cost containment has decreased the time physicians can provide for caring and compassion. The pressures to make physicians into entrepreneurs risk the loss of their commitment to the primacy of patient needs.

Implicit in the allocation of the task of caring for the health of citizens is the obligation of society, either through the state, the corporate sector, charitable organizations, or a combination of them all, to provide sufficient resources so that individual physicians can meet their responsibilities to patients and that the profession collectively may meet its obligations to society. One way of examining how different countries have met these obligations is by calculating the percentage of the gross domestic product (GDP) that they allocate to health care. For many years the United Kingdom devoted a lower percentage of its GDP to health services than the Organization for Economic Cooperation and Development (OECD) average, and public dissatisfaction forced the government to attempt to narrow the gap by adding significantly to the funds devoted to health. Cost cutting in Canada in the 1990s led to an under-resourced health-care system, and pressure from both the medical profession and the general public led to a partial refunding of the system. The strong voice of the profession, acting through the Canadian Medical Association in renegotiating the social contract, was both appropriate and effective.

The United States, which in modern times has led the world in health-care expenditures, certainly cannot be accused of devoting insufficient resources to health care. However, the presence of a significant percentage of the population who are uninsured can be interpreted as an indication that society is failing to meet its obligations to some of its citizens. The lack of resources makes it extraordinarily difficult for physicians, who must function within a system that does not allow them to provide adequate care to a subset of the population.

If a contract that preserves the values of the healer and the professional is to be maintained, those representing the profession must convince society that it is in society's interests to have a system based upon justice and equity, as well as one that is adequately funded, no matter what the structure of the health-care system. This is a legitimate expectation, not only of the medical profession, but of individual citizens.

Autonomy

Autonomy has been described by some sociologists as the hallmark of a profession.[30] Thus, under the contract, physicians expect to be granted sufficient freedom in practice that they may act in the best interests of their patients. This autonomy has never been unlimited. Custom, codes of ethics, and legal constraints have limited it. However, the ability of a physician, in collaboration with a patient, to determine a proper course of action remains sacrosanct to the practice of medicine. If the medical profession feels that it is no longer able to act in the best interest of its patients, it can legitimately resist unreasonable intrusions into its autonomy and can insist on the maintenance of conditions that will ensure that it is able to carry out its assigned task of serving patients. Unwarranted intrusions such as gag laws have been deemed to be unacceptable, and it is significant that both the profession and society rejected them. Second opinions and clinical guidelines, while perhaps resented when rigidly applied, have been deemed to be reasonable for establishing standards of care. As the system evolves, sufficient autonomy remains important to the profession.

Trust

In spite of the failings of some individual physicians and of the perception that medicine's organizations may have favored the interests of their own members over the public good, medicine remains among the most trusted occupations, and its practitioners' incomes remain high in most countries. Most physicians demonstrate morality and integrity, work to remain competent, and carry out their activities to the best of their abilities while demonstrating concern for the welfare of their patients. They believe that this should be recognized and that they deserve the trust of those they serve. Contemporary physicians are more concerned about lack of trust than they are about the details of practice or financial matters.[31] They appear to believe that society is not meeting its legitimate expectations and is misinformed. To quote an eminent sociologist: "Professionalism is based on the real character of certain services, it is not a clever invention of selfish minds."[32] Medicine must convince society by its conduct that this is correct, because physicians clearly believe that maintaining trust is important to healing.

Status and Rewards

Through the ages, the healer and the professional have received both financial and nonfinancial rewards from society. In fact, before the practice of medicine became as lucrative as it did during the twentieth century, the nonfinancial aspects were perhaps more important.[33] Status in the community and the respect of fellow citizens were important aspects of the attractiveness of medicine as a career, and they remain an expectation of physicians. It is also evident that contemporary physicians expect to receive reasonable remuneration for their services, and they do. Medicine remains one of the best-paid occupations.

Recent changes in the health-care systems, and hence in the social contract, have caused physicians to question their treatment by society, and it appears that changes in the nonfinancial parts of the contract—trust, status and respect—are of more concern than are financial matters.[34]

Monopoly

The modern profession of medicine dates from the middle of the nineteenth century, when licensing laws granted physicians the exclusive right to prac-

tice medicine.[35] Prior to that time, the healing arts were essentially unregu-
lated, and allopathic medicine competed (sometimes not very effectively)
with alternative forms of healing. Although many activities that were previously considered to be exclusive to the practice of medicine have been
taken over by nurses, physician's assistants, and other health-care professionals, medicine has maintained a monopoly over its core activities.

As one looks into the future, one can safely predict that this trend will grow
but that medicine will continue to control the central activities of the diagnosis and treatment of human disease. As it is determined that other health-care
professionals are competent to carry out a group of procedures, modern science will add others to medicine's monopoly. Medicine's attitude in
approaching this issue should clearly be determined by what is best for the
patient and society, rather than being overprotective of its jurisdiction. Placing the public good first is a professional obligation and part of the social
contract. However, medicine can legitimately expect that the core activities
of a physician will continue to be protected by licensing laws.

Self-Regulation

The modern medical profession was granted the privilege of self-regulation
as part of the social contract.[36] The complexity of medicine's knowledge base
and of the practice of medicine is the principal justification for self-regulation. Because of this complexity it is difficult, but not impossible, for the state
to regulate the practice of medicine. Where state regulation does take place,
as in France, physicians are utilized to actually develop and carry out the
activity under guidelines established in law.[37] While self-regulation has been
questioned, in large part because of medicine's failures, it has generally been
concluded that it has advantages to society. However, when the profession
fails to carry out its duties to the satisfaction of society, the contract may be
altered, and the state may repatriate some self-regulatory activities, as has
happened recently in Britain.[38] Thus, medicine's obligation to self-regulate,
and to be regarded as doing this well, becomes doubly important. This has
been an area of intense negotiations in many parts of the world as accountability in economic and political terms has become expected. In essence,
medicine's expectations under the contract have often clashed with societal
expectations. In the future, medicine must maintain ways to listen to society's
expectations and to negotiate a satisfactory response.

SUMMARY AND CONCLUSIONS

A tacit agreement does exist between medicine and society, which has been
termed a "social contract." Because society has chosen to use the concept of

the profession as a means of organizing the services of the healer, professionalism has come to serve as the basis of medicine's social contract. Essential portions of what is expected of the physician as healer are determined by what it means to be a professional in contemporary society. It is incumbent upon the medical profession to understand professionalism and the obligations that are necessary to sustain it because these serve as the basis for societal expectations. It is also necessary for those representing society to understand both the presence and the nature of the contract and society's obligations under it.

Two points should be emphasized. First, the social contract requires that the medical profession be trusted. Physicians must also have trust in the fairness of the health-care system, or they may cease to act in a professional way, with unfortunate consequences for the system.[39] It is therefore important to both parties to maintain high levels of trust. Second, unreasonable expectations by either side can lead to disillusionment and a loss of trust. For example, for a physician at any level to be on call too often in the name of altruism is unreasonable, as is a medical profession that demands resources that are deemed excessive by society. The contract can only function properly if each side agrees to meet the reasonable expectations of the other.

NOTES

1. J. W. Gough, *The Social Contract: A Critical Study of Its Development* (Oxford: Clarendon Press, 1957).

2. P. Starr, *The Social Transformation of American Medicine* (New York: Basic Books, 1984); W. Sullivan, *Work and integrity: The Crisis and Promise of Professionalism in North America* (New York: Harper Collins, 1995); E. Krause, *Death of the Guilds: Professions, States and the Advance of Capitalism, 1930 to the Present* (New Haven, CT: Yale University Press, 1996); J. A. Barondess, "Medicine and Professionalism," *Archives of Internal Medicine* 163 (2003): 1–15; S. R. Cruess and R. L. Cruess, "Professionalism: A Contract between Medicine and Society," *Canadian Medical Association Journal* 162 (2000): 668–69.

3. R. L. Cruess and S. R. Cruess, "Teaching Medicine as a Profession in the Service of Healing," *Academic Medicine* 72 (1997): 941–52.

4. D. Mechanic, "Changing Medical Organization and the Erosion of Trust," *Milbank Quarterly* 74 (1996): 171–89.

5. L. Gilson, "Trust and the Development of Health Care as a Social Institution," *Social Science and Medicine* 56 (2003): 1453–68.

6. Krause, *Death of the Guilds;* M. A. Schlesinger, "Loss of Faith: The Sources of Reduced Political Legitimacy for the American Medical Profession," *Milbank Quarterly* 80 (2002): 185–235; A. Zuger, "Dissatisfaction with Medical Practice," *New England Journal of Medicine* 350 (2004): 69–75.

7. Starr, *The Social Transformation;* E. Freidson, *Professional Dominance: The Social Structure of Medical Care* (Chicago: Aldine, 1970); M. Larson, *The Rise of Professionalism: A Sociological Analysis* (Berkeley and Los Angeles: University of California Press, 1977).

8. Starr, *The Social Transformation.*

9. Gough, *The Social Contract,* 245.

10. T. Brennan et al., "Medical Professionalism in the New Millennium: A Physician's Charter," *Lancet* 359 (2002): 520–22, and *Annals of Internal Medicine* 136 (2002): 243–46.

11. Cruess and Cruess, "Teaching Medicine as a Profession."

12. E. D. Pellegrino and A. Relman, "Professional Medical Associations: Ethical and Practical Guidelines," *Journal of the American Medical Association* 282 (1999): 1954–56.

13. Zuger, "Dissatisfaction with Medical Practice."

14. R. Stevens, "Public Roles for the Medical Profession in the United States: Beyond Theories of Decline and Fall," *Milbank Quarterly* 79 (2001): 327–53.

15. Zuger, "Dissatisfaction with Medical Practice"; Pellegrino and Relman, "Professional Medical Associations."

16. L. Brandeis, *Business: A Profession* (Boston: Hale, Cushman and Flint, 1933).

17. R. L. Gruen, S. D. Pearson, and T. A. Brennan, "Physician-Citizens: Public Roles and Professional Obligations," *Journal of the American Medical Association* 291 (2004): 94–98.

18. Starr, *The Social Transformation;* Krause, *Death of the Guilds.*

19. Gough, *The Social Contract;* Sullivan, *Work and Integrity;* Freidson, *Professional Dominance.*

20. Larson, *The Rise of Professionalism.*

21. E. J. Emanuel and L. L. Emanuel, "What Is Accountability in Health Care?" *Annals of Internal Medicine* 124 (1996): 229–39.

22. Pellegrino and Relman, "Professional Medical Associations."

23. Emanuel and Emanuel, "What Is Accountability in Health Care?"

24. Gruen, Pearson, and Brennan, "Physician-Citizens."

25. B. E. Landon, J. Reschovsky, and D. Blumenthal, "Changes in Career Satisfaction among Primary Care and Specialist Physicians, 1977–2001," *Journal of the American Medical Association* 289 (2003): 442–49; B. Sibbald, C. Bojke, and H. Gravelle, "National Survey of Job Satisfaction and Retirement Intentions among General Practitioners in England," *British Medical Journal* 326 (2003): 22–24.

26. M. K. Wynia, S. R Latham, A. C. Kao, J. W. Berg, and L. L. Emanuel, "Medical Professionalism in Society," *New England Journal of Medicine* 341 (1999): 1612–16.

27. D. Pendleton and J. King, "Values and Leadership," *British Medical Journal* 325 (2002): 1352–55.

28. D. W. Light, "The Medical Profession and Organizational Change: From Professional Dominance to Countervailing Power," in *Handbook of Medical Sociology,* eds. C. E. Bird, P. Conrad, and A. M. Fremont, 201–16, 5th ed. (Upper Saddle River, NJ: Prentice Hall, 2000).

29. M. Moran and B. Wood. *States, Regulation and the Medical Profession* (Buckingham, UK: Open University Press, 1993).

30. Freidson, *Professional Dominance.*

31. Landon, Reschovsky, and Blumenthal, "Changes in Career Satisfaction"; Sibbald, Bojke, and Gravelle, "National Survey of Job Satisfaction."

32. T. H. Marshall, "The Recent History of Professionalism in Relation to Social Structure and Social Policy," *Canadian Journal of Economics and Political Science* 15 (1939): 325–40.

33. Gough, *The Social Contract;* Sullivan, *Work and Integrity.*

34. Zuger, "Dissatisfaction with Medical Practice."

35. Gough, *The Social Contract;* Sullivan, *Work and Integrity.*

36. Starr, *The Social Transformation;* Sullivan, *Work and Integrity;*

37. Sullivan, *Work and Integrity.*

38. R. Smith, "All Changed, Changed Utterly: British Medicine Will Be Transformed by the Bristol Case," *British Medical Journal* 316 (1998): 1917–18.

39. D. Blumenthal, "The Vital Role of Professionalism in Health Care Reform," *Health Affairs* 13 (1994): 252–56.

3

The Birth of Medical Professionalism: Professionalism and the Role of Professional Associations

Matthew Wynia

For most of recorded history, until the advent of the American Medical Association (AMA) in 1847, there was no such thing as the "medical profession."

Today, this reads like a very bold assertion indeed. As the proportion of doctors who are members of the AMA has fallen, and the organization's influence among policy makers may be in decline,[1] some readers might find it hard to believe that this same organization, the structure of which has changed very little since its foundation, actually created the very notion of medicine as a profession. Yet in 1847 the founding of the AMA and the promulgation of its *Code of Medical Ethics* were widely recognized as revolutionary and as having international sociocultural as well as medical implications. As Baker, Caplan, Emanuel, and Latham have observed, the AMA *Code* was "the world's first national code of *professional* ethics, the world's first national code of *medical* ethics, and the ancestor of all professional codes of ethics, medical or nonmedical. In its time, the AMA *Code* was a revolutionary document that was thought to be comparable to the Declaration of Independence."[2] Revolutionary concepts that were first collected together in the AMA *Code*—such as professional self-regulation; reciprocal obligations of professionals to patients, society, and each other; obedience of individual professionals to rules of practice established by one's peers; collective duties of self-sacrifice in service to those seeking one's help—have become familiar elements of all professions and occupations that aspire to professionalization. They were not so prior to 1847.

OATHS, CODES, AND COLLECTIVE
MEDICAL ETHICS

To be sure, from the time of Hippocrates and even before, there were many treatises on what we might now call medical ethics—essays on why physicians should provide charity care, seek excellence in practice, and in general be gentlemen of honor and virtue. Some ethical standards derived from religion, which was very important to physicians; illness and sin were often thought to be linked, and healing for a time was closely associated with the priesthood.[3] And, of course, there was the Hippocratic oath itself—the most famous and enduring personal pledge taken by physicians to act in certain ways and to benefit, or at least not intentionally harm, one's patients. There had been some licensure requirements for medical practice, at least as far back as 1231 in Italy, and physicians of the Holy Roman Empire were sometimes sued for malpractice.[4] Yet these elements and others had never been brought together in a cohesive whole to fulfill what we now conceive of as a "profession." Professions, after all, are not defined merely by whether a practitioner can be sued—they have specific social roles and expectations, they seek explicitly, *as a group*, to ensure that every member of the profession lives up to these expectations, and hence they have formal structures for self-regulation.

In addition to the absence of certain social constructs (namely, near-universal membership in a professional association that can set rules for practice, to which we shall return shortly), it has also been argued that there was no coherent ethical construct in which to place the obligations of "medical professionals" (or any other professionals, for that matter) until the creation of the AMA *Code of Medical Ethics*. The *Code* contained the first set of specific and widely recognized expectations that were to be applied to every American physician—and in exchange for the profession's assurance that all its practitioners live up to these expectations, society and individual patients were said to hold reciprocal obligations toward medical professionals. This notion of reciprocity, so central to the 1847 AMA *Code*, had its roots in social contract theory (the origins of which extend as far back as Plato's *Republic*, and in the philosophical writings of Hobbes, Locke, Rousseau, Hume, and others).[5] But the use of reciprocity as the foundation for professional obligations and rights was particularly well suited (at the time) to certain uniquely American sensibilities. Specifically, setting professional obligations as part of a social contract implicitly acknowledged that being a good doctor did not require that one come from the gentlemanly classes. Good doctors could come from any class, as long as they were well trained, scientifically competent, and aware of all their specified obligations. Furthermore, because

Americans had adopted a unique form of liberal democratic values, it was also uniquely American to assert that the nature of social interactions and governance ought to be based on mutual agreement rather than the assertion of raw power. That is, medical professionals were to retain their social standing and privileges not because they had gained powerful positions, but because they would keep the promises they had made.

It is important to recognize that social contracts, like codes of ethics, are not the same as oaths. Traditionally, oaths like the Hippocratic oath are a personal promise of virtuous behavior made to the gods ("I swear, by Apollo Physician and Asclepius and Hygieia and Panaceia and all the gods and goddesses, making them my witnesses, that I will fulfill according to my ability and judgment this oath and this covenant"). Codes of ethics, by contrast, are based on a fully collective, almost impersonal ethic, one premised on the group's adherence to a set of explicit promises to society regarding, for example, competence, self-sacrifice, and self-control. Hence, the 1847 *Code of Medical Ethics* did not much rely on appeals to personal virtue or to a deity. Instead it accepted, and even promoted, the idea that a claim of "professionalism" entails taking on a special social role, as laid out in the code, with clearly delineated obligations to patients, the community, and other professionals. Indeed, under this conception of professionalism, it could be said that the primary necessary personal virtue of physicians is that they hold interprofessional relations at a premium, because it is interprofessional relations that form the bedrock of a coherent profession.

In sum, although U.S. physicians after 1847 were certainly expected to be genteel, this was not expected to come from noble breeding or religion, as it had in the past, but instead from physicians' adherence to an explicit contractual relationship. This social contract was drawn up by doctors themselves as the AMA *Code of Medical Ethics*, which derived its force from 1) its uniform application among all physicians, and 2) the reciprocal and specific obligations and rights it afforded to patients, society, and physicians. In two respects, then, one can say that although there had been the concept of a "good doctor" prior to 1847, there had been no such thing as a good medical professional. First, prior to 1847 there had been no coherent set of rules and structures in any nation that applied to all physicians regarding training, competence, and obligations of social service. The AMA was established specifically to provide such rules and the structures necessary for maintaining them. Second, there had been no coherent ethical grounding for such structures and rules to take hold. The AMA *Code* was explicitly based in the notion of a social contract and relied on the ethical construct of reciprocity.

It is a reflection of this "birth" of medical professionalism that it was only after "the American medical ethics revolution" of 1847 that social scientists could, and did, begin to explore the meaning and role of medical professionals in society.

THE STRUCTURAL FUNCTIONALISTS

In the early part of the twentieth century, consistent with the conceptions of contract and reciprocity laid out in the AMA *Code*, medical professionalism was understood according to the structuralist-functionalist school of the sociologist Talcott Parsons and his students.[6] This approach listed distinctive characteristics of professional groups and sought to discern the socially desirable rationales for each characteristic. That is, it asked, what does society get in exchange for each specific professional obligation or right? For example, medical professionals tend to take obligations of confidentiality very seriously, because this allows patients to disclose sensitive information—such as about infectious disease exposures—that might prove useful to society in halting the spread of disease. Medical professionals value cooperation rather than competition with each other, because this speeds dissemination of new knowledge.[7] Professionals are allowed largely to self-regulate, because their work is complex and fluid, requiring constant full-time exposure—that is, "practice"—to enable competent oversight of other practitioners.

When these sociologists considered why physicians might not follow their own selfish interests and maximize profits by taking advantage of sick patients, Parsons and his followers postulated that physicians did, indeed, follow selfish interests—but fortunately for society, physicians' self-interests tended to lie less in making money than in improving one's status amongst one's peers.[8] That is, professionals place a very high value on collegial interactions; this explains why professional associations were so important to the birth and maintenance of professionalism.

An effective social contract relies on the existence of a cohesive group to create and enforce it. Near-universal membership in the AMA at the turn of the century and for decades thereafter provided this necessary structure. By the turn of the century, virtually every well-regarded and successful physician was an active member of numerous professional groups, the most important of which was the AMA. Even in the wilderness of the west, collegial interactions were highly valued, and physicians would travel long distances, at some risk, to discuss work with their peers and to learn new techniques. It was proposed that physicians could remain competent only through participation in organized professional associations, because only there could they exchange information, share experiences that those outside the profession would not understand (or appreciate), and even rebuke each other for poor practice.

Perhaps the most famous example of such a physician leader is Sir William Osler, who was called an "organization man" for his involvement in more than one hundred different professional organizations.[9] Indeed, Osler espoused the notion that membership in professional organizations, even unrelated to any personal gains that might accrue from membership, was an obligation for physicians. He declared that "no physician has a right to consider himself as belonging to himself; but all ought to regard themselves as belonging to the profession, inasmuch as each is a part of the profession."[10] He also asserted, "You cannot afford to stand aloof from your professional colleagues in any place. Join their associations, mingle in their meetings, gathering here, scattering there; but everywhere showing that you are faithful students, as willing to teach as be taught."[11] Once, when asked by a medical student what he, the student, would get out of attending a medical society meeting, Osler replied, "Do you think I attend for what I can get out of it, or for what I can put into it?"[12]

THE CRITICAL POWER THEORISTS

What might be called the era of organized medicine, after more than one hundred years of ascendancy, began to decline in the 1960s, as the structuralist-functionalist conception of the professions came under vigorous attack by Eliot Freidson and his followers, including the prominent sociologist Paul Starr, in the 1980s. While organized medicine would continue to wield great social power throughout the 1960s and into the 1970s, the groundwork for its decline was laid in the remarkably influential work of this new school of academic sociologists, who were called "critical power theorists." This school of thought saw the structural functionalists as naive and strongly suspected that professionals were not as altruistic as had been claimed, and they collected data and historical anecdotes to support this assertion.[13] Some critics starkly challenged physicians' ethics, claiming that professional ethics were largely a "cynical ploy" to create, and then profit from, monopoly power in the market.[14]

Interestingly, some of these sociologists (most notably Freidson) have subsequently reasserted the value of medical professionalism, including self-regulation and the norms created through codes of ethics,[15] in light of subsequent experience with the rising power of marketplace values in medical care. But the fundamental criticisms of the power theorists remain very influential and commonly held by academic sociologists. Most importantly, these cri-

tiques—aimed primarily at disproving physician claims of altruism and to
some extent competence—underlay landmark legal actions against physicians under the antitrust statutes.[16] Professional associations, and the AMA
in particular, were told by the courts that setting professional standards could
be tantamount to restraint of trade and the creation of monopoly power. And
so, for example, under court order the AMA was forced to alter its code of
ethics in 1980 to allow most forms of advertising for physician services.[17] Of
course, the notion that professional associations can and should create and
enforce standards for practice *is* a type of restraint of trade—the purpose of
which is to lock irregular, and potentially dangerous, practitioners out of the
practice of medicine, which is a service to the public. But the courts did not
see the professional associations as wielding this power to restrain trade
responsibly—hence it was, in part, taken away.

TECHNOLOGY, AUTONOMY, AND CHANGING
NOTIONS OF PROFESSIONALISM

Remarkably, physicians in the 1980s did not uniformly fight this trend—
some were in fact delighted to be able to advertise, and not all mourned the
loss of AMA power—in part because many physicians' conceptions of professionalism were changing. These changes came in several related technological, sociological, and ethical ways.

With regard to technology, the extremely rapid rise in useful diagnostic
and treatment methods fed growing beliefs that medical professionals derived
their social standing from their special training and the ability to harness technology rather than from any social contract rooted in civic obligations. This
sense of professionalism as grounded solely in technical competence, though
understandable, would lead to both a declining sense of social mission among
physicians as well as poor "'customer service'" values. After all, if one can
offer lifesaving therapy, other facets of customer service might seem to pale
in comparison. There is a connection among physicians' excessive reliance
on technology, poor customer service, and medical paternalism, which contributed to the backlash against professional authority in the 1970s and later.
And all these factors were buttressed by additional trends that contributed
to the notion that physicians are self-interested rather than altruistic or civic
minded.

First, especially after 1912, organized medicine had perceived the possibility of government intervention in medical care as a major threat. Thus, for
example, in 1957 the AMA *Code* proclaimed bluntly that it is a primary ethical principle that "a physician may choose whom to serve."[18] Second, with

this growing emphasis on individual physician autonomy, the common understanding of "professional autonomy" mutated. With the evolving sense that professionalism meant the ability of each doctor to treat patients as they wanted, there developed a conflation between classical professional autonomy (the right of the group to self-regulate) and personal autonomy (the right of individual members to do as they please). Hence, while professionalism had been born around the notion that the group would set and enforce shared standards, it came to be construed as granting individual physicians the right to choose how to treat each patient. In effect, "professionalism" came to be understood, wrongly, as a license to practice without meaningful oversight.

Finally, medical ethics increasingly stressed the importance of autonomy as a principle, de-emphasizing both physicians' and patients' social obligations.[19] Consistent with this strong focus on individual autonomy, many medical ethicists urged physicians to ignore civic considerations altogether and think only of the welfare of the individual patient before them. For instance, in 1984 Dr. Norman Levinsky wrote, "Physicians are required to do everything that they believe may benefit each patient, without regard to costs or other societal considerations."[20] Such a statement reflects the domination of medical ethics by respect for individual autonomy, but it also illustrates the loss of a cardinal facet of the social contract that had grounded physician professionalism, which Parsons had described: mediation between private and community interests.[21]

PROFESSIONS AS SOCIAL MEDIATORS

Parsons had claimed that medical professionals serve as part of the social fabric, acting as "interstitial go-betweens" by helping to reintegrate ill persons into society. In essence, physicians are granted powers to protect the ill (such as by allowing time off work or granting disabled parking permits) in exchange for a collective promise to help society by working to return the ill to productive life. To play this role, it is important that physicians serve neither the patient nor the community alone—hence the need for professional autonomy with strong collegial oversight.[22] Physicians earn patients' trust by promising to look out for their best interests, but they earn the social right to do so by promising society that they will, as a group, take seriously their civic roles. This balancing act is not easy, but it is core to the effective functioning of medical professionalism in society.

Wynia and Gostin note that medicine since the 1950s, having largely abandoned its "role as a social protector, has been left with only technical expertise to support its claims to professional prerogatives, which are granted by society and which have since steadily eroded."[23] Others have also recognized this chain of events, and many recent scholars of the medical profession suggest that a civic understanding of professionalism is necessary to maintain public trust.[24]

THE DECLINING ROLE OF PROFESSIONAL ASSOCIATIONS

With the decline in the understanding of professionalism as governing a social contract, the social standing of professional associations, which are charged with writing this contract, has declined.[25] Membership in many professional associations is down, especially in the state and national groups that focus on shared social issues. On the other hand, reflecting the conception of professionalism as focused on technical competence, membership in clinical subspecialty associations remains high. Indeed, most physicians still belong to three or more professional groups, though fewer than one-third are members of the AMA.

But what is the role of the AMA and other multispecialty societies, such as state medical associations, if specialty societies provide technical competence, and there is no clear social contract or self-regulatory function for the broader associations? The role of contemporary national professional associations can be understood best in relation to alternative methods for organizing the delivery of health-care services. Modern medical care is of sufficient social value that ensuring its quality is important for a well-functioning society. But if professional associations are not empowered to establish and enforce norms of practice, then another mechanism would need to be used to ensure the quality of medical care. Apart from professional self-regulation, two options exist: quality might be regulated through the marketplace, or it might be regulated according to governmental rule making and enforcement. Both options have their proponents, but it suffices for our purposes to note that as the power of professional associations has waned, U.S. health care has applied both methods in various degrees to a variety of situations.

MARKETS AND CONSUMERISM IN MEDICAL CARE

Markets are sometimes said to follow no ethical norms, but this is not the case. A well-functioning market demands strict adherence to rules of truth telling. That is, markets function effectively only when all participants are well-informed. Since this is also a primary value in health care (even in ancient times it was recognized that a well-informed and participatory patient is more likely to adhere to therapy and hence to improve),[26] this suggests that health care might be well served in a free market. On the other hand, there are some situations when it is not possible for patients to act as informed consumers, such as emergency situations and when illness clouds judgment. In addition, classical free markets also require easy entry and exit for both buyers and sellers, known and stable preferences of buyers, no externalities associated with the good being sold (that is, whether or not a buyer chooses to buy has no effect on other potential buyers), and no information asymmetry (sellers don't know more about the product than buyers do, or vice versa).[27] It has become a truism that these classic requirements for an effective free market are rarely, if ever, met in health-care settings.

MEDICAL CARE AND THE STATE

If markets are only partially effective in ensuring the efficient delivery of high-quality health care, then perhaps state controls are more attractive. Indeed, outside the United States, health care has generally come to be seen as a human right that should be guaranteed, in some degree, by the state. This view of health care may be prudential (a healthy population is a more productive population), based in norms of morality, or both. Regardless, in the United States there has been much less agreement that health care should be treated like education, clean air and water, and other social goods (also called "common goods") from which all citizens derive benefit and toward the provision of which the state therefore has obligations.

While greater levels of state regulation appear to have worked acceptably well in other countries, many—perhaps even the majority—of Americans are not convinced. Some argue that state-based regulation of health care might lead to reduced innovation. Others worry that governmental allocation of resources would be inappropriately utilitarian and could lead to unacceptable rationing of health care and loss of autonomy for patients and physicians. While proponents of greater governmental involvement dispute these assertions, these ongoing debates show few signs of near-term resolution.

BRIDGING THE GAPS

Fortunately, movement forward does not require full resolution of the long-standing argument over whether to orient the health-care system more toward markets (which foster innovation but exclude those who cannot pay) or more toward governmental regulation (which can ensure universal coverage but can be inappropriately utilitarian and stifle incentives for innovation). Indeed, it is the proper role of medical professional associations to help society bridge this gap. Just as Parsons noted that individual professionals serve as a bridge between ill people and their communities, professional associations should serve, ideally, to moderate the potentially negative effects of both markets and governmental regulation within health care.

For example, while one can make an idealized case for organizing a health-care system using only marketplace, governmental, or professional mechanisms, in reality all three mechanisms are used, often in combination. Markets are regulated by governments (though not as much as some would like) to ensure fair play. Governmental support for care of the poor, disabled, and elderly is vast, though experiments with market methods are being tried in these domains as well. Governmental regulatory functions are informed by professional standards. Legal standards for malpractice are informed by professional association standards, guidelines, and codes of ethics. In a few states, the AMA *Code of Medical Ethics* is incorporated directly into state medical practice laws. Members of state medical boards are frequently appointed by state medical societies, which have a hand in setting licensure requirements. Accrediting organizations such as the Joint Commission on Accreditation of Health Care Organizations (JCAHO) have been created specifically to use all three methods. JCAHO requirements (quality standards set by professionals) are used as criteria for receipt of state-based financing (a state regulatory structure) and also to empower patients to choose higher-quality health-care providers (a market mechanism to drive health-care quality). Indeed, some might argue that a profession's success is defined by the degree to which the profession's self-regulatory structures become sanctioned by the state, making professional self-regulation and state regulation inextricably intertwined.

At the same time, however, it is critical that professions, and professional associations, maintain some distance from the state and the market. For different reasons, the state and market both tend not to protect the most vulnerable among us, despite the fact that doing so is critical to a just society. As noted above, markets are not structured to serve the interests of the impoverished ill, while state policies, of necessity, tend toward a utilitarian cost-benefit calculus that can ultimately victimize the human rights of vulnerable populations. In the end, this is the social role of the organizations physicians have formed to maintain our profession. Our profession and our professional associations exist, not for the benefit of medical professionals, but for the benefit of the communities and the vulnerable patients we serve.

NOTES

1. M. A. Schlesinger, "Loss of Faith: The Sources of Reduced Political Legitimacy for the American Medical Profession," *Milbank Quarterly* 80 (2002): 185–235.

2. R. B. Baker, A. L. Caplan, L. L. Emanuel, and S. R. Latham, eds., *The American Medical Ethics Revolution: How the AMA's Code of Ethics Has Transformed Physicians' Relationships to Patients, Professionals, and Society* (Baltimore: Johns Hopkins University Press, 1999).

3. K. E. Geraghty and M. K. Wynia, "Advocacy and Community: The Social Role of Physicians over the Last 1,000 Years," part 1, *Medscape General Medicine,* October 30, 2000, www.medscape.com/Medscape/GeneralMedicine/journal/2000/v02.n05/mgm1030 .gera/mgm1030.gera-01.html.

4. A. Jonsen, "Hellenic, Hellenistic, and Roman Medicine," in *A Short History of Medical Ethics* (New York: Oxford University Press, 2000).

5. Perhaps the earliest mention of a social contract is in Plato's *Republic*, in which Glaucon notes that "men decide they would be better off if they made a compact neither to do wrong nor to suffer it. Hence they began to make laws and covenants with one another." For more on the history of social contracts, see Social Contract, in *The Dictionary of the History of Ideas,* etext.lib.virginia.edu/cgi-local/DHI/dhi.cgi?id = dv4-34 (accessed February 6, 2004).

6. T. Parsons, "The Professions and Social Structure," *Social Forces* 17 (1939): 45–67.

7. There were to be no trade secrets among honorable professionals. Indeed, the AMA roundly condemned "patent medicine" and stimulated the formation of the Food and Drug Administration to close dishonorable practitioners out of the profession.

8. S. R. Latham, "Medical Professionalism: A Parsonian View," *Mt. Sinai Journal of Medicine* 69 (6): 363–69.

9. W. Olser, "The Army Surgeon," in *Aequanimitas. With other Addresses to Medical Students, Nurses, and Practitioners of Medicine* (Philadelphia: P Blakiston's Son, 1932).

10. W. Osler, "The Functions of a State Faculty," *Maryland Medical Journal* 37 (1897): 73–77.

11. C. S. Bryan, *Osler: Inspirations from a Great Physician* (New York: Oxford University Press, 1997).

12. Olser, "The Army Surgeon."

13. P. Starr, *The Social Transformation of American Medicine* (New York: Basic Books, 1982).

14. Osler, "The Functions of a State Faculty."

15. E. Freidson, *Professionalism Reborn: Theory, Prophecy and Policy* (Chicago: University of Chicago Press, 1994).

16. R. Curry, "AMA vs. FTC," in *Medicine for Sale* (Knoxville, TN: Grand Rounds Press, 1992).

17. American Medical Association, *Code of Medical Ethics* (Chicago: AMA Press, 2004), opinion 5.02, advertising and publicity.

18. Judicial Council, American Medical Association. Principles of Medical Ethics. June 7, 1958. Available at: www.ama-assn.org/ama/upload/mm/369/1957_principles.pdf (accessed April 8, 2006).

19. W. M. Sage, "Physicians as Advocates," *Houston Law Review* 35 (1999): 1529–630; A. I. Applebaum, *Ethics for Adversaries* (Princeton, NJ: Princeton University Press, 1999).

20. N. Levinsky, "The Doctor's Master," *New England Journal of Medicine* 311 (1984): 1573–75.

21. Parsons, "The Professions and Social Structure."

22. Properly understood, professional autonomy is not so much a defining feature of professionalism as a simple necessity for physicians to best carry out their social role. The fact that Parsons and his students looked at professional autonomy as a defining feature, rather than a necessary characteristic, of professionalism may have facilitated the subsequent criticism that claims to professional autonomy were a cynical ploy and counter to the public good.

23. M. K. Wynia and L. O. Gostin, "Ethical Challenges in Preparing for Bioterrorism: The Role of the Health Care System," *American Journal of Public Health* (July, 2004) 94 (7):1096–102.

24. W. M. Sullivan, "What Is Left of Professionalism after Managed Care?" *Hasting Center Report* 29 (1999): 7–13; Schlesinger, "Loss of Faith"; H. M. Swick, "Toward a Normative Definition of Medical Professionalism," *Academic Medicine* 75 (2000): 612–16; Latham, "Medical Professionalism."

25. Schlesinger, "Loss of Faith."

26. Plato wrote of "slave medicine," wherein "the physician never gives the slave any account of his complaints, nor asks for any," as contrasted with medicine for free men, in which "the physician treats their disease by going into things thoroughly from the beginning in a scientific way and takes the patient and his family into confidence. Thus he learns something from the patients. He never gives prescriptions until he has won the patient's support, and when he has done so, he aims to produce complete restoration to health by persuading the patient to comply." Plato, *The Laws*, quoted in M. Siegler, "Lessons from 30 Years of Teaching Clinical Ethics," *Virtual Mentor,* October 2001, www.ama-assn.org/ama/pub/category/6557.html (accessed March 10, 2006).

27. L. C. Thurow, "Medicine versus Economics," *New England Journal of Medicine* 313 (10) (1985): 611–14.

4

Professionalism and Commercialism as Antitheticals: A Search for "Unprofessional Commercialism" within the Writings and Work of American Medicine

Frederic W. Hafferty

The call to place the patient's welfare above all other enjoinments has been a core element in medicine's march to professionhood. Issues of commercialism have been a historical part of this record—witness this excerpt from the prayer of Maimonides: "inspire me with love for my art and for Thy creatures. Do not allow thirst for profit, ambition for renown and admiration, to interfere with my profession, for these are the enemies of truth and of love for mankind." As medicine evolved, it was enjoined organizationally to structure the delivery of health-care services, including aspects of organizational culture, so that they supported and helped to put into operation this most fundamental of tenets. Enjoinders and obligations, however, can be distorted as the modern medical corporation subverts traditional values to rhetoric and advertisements ("the patient, above all else"). Even what one considers a commodity has changed. In today's medicine, commercial transactions not only include traditional goods and services but also the sale of patients themselves, as companies battle for "market territory," and "covered lives." While today's public understands that physicians must charge for their services, it is difficult for this same public to appreciate the myriad of ways in which the commodification of medicine has come to influence behaviors that are directed more toward the enrichment of individual practitioners, corporations, and stockholders than toward patient welfare. Although the commercialization of medicine has been denounced time and again by medical leaders,[1] it remains unclear whether these warnings have had a transformative effect on the shop floor and/or in the boardrooms of modern medicine.

The thesis of this chapter is that organized medicine's denunciation of commercialism in medicine is fundamentally self-serving and essentially shallow unless it translates these denunciations into standards that are in turn employed and enforced in the service of patients. The physician-patient relationship remains the hub of medicine's social contract with society.[2] This is where medicine affirms, or fails, in its insistence that "patient primacy" is the core medical value.[3] Failure to affirm and enforce the primacy of patient welfare in general, and in the face of commercial pressures in particular, risks that the profession and its practitioners will lose the public's trust and that medicine will slide from being a revered profession to an occupation populated with technical experts.

Does organized medicine acknowledge the threat of commercialism and put disciplinary muscle in defining and punishing unprofessional behavior related to conflicts between profit and patient? To answer this question, we will work through four related exercises. First, we will consider two examples of physician commercialism, both taken from public news reports. Second, using these examples, we will examine six contemporary statements of medicine's professional and ethical core and consider how commercialism and its threats to medical professionalism are defined and addressed. These six codes are 1) the American Medical Association's (AMA) *Principles of Medical Ethics (revised in 2001)*; 2) the AMA *Declaration of Professional Responsibility: Medicine's Social Contract with Humanity*; 3) the AMA *Code of Medical Ethics: Current Opinions with Annotations (2004 edition)*; 4) the American College of Physicians' *Ethics Manual (Fourth edition)*, 5) the Federation of State Medical Boards' *Guide to the Essentials of Modern Medical Practice (Tenth edition)*, with particular attention to the section "Disciplinary Action Against Licensees: Grounds for Action," and, finally, 6) the *Medical Professionalism in the New Millennium: A Physician Charter*, a collaborative effort by the members of the American Board of Internal Medicine Federation (ABIM), the American College of Physicians–American Society of Internal Medicine (ACP-ASIM), and the European Federation of Internal Medicine. As our third exercise, we will visit the Web sites of several state medical boards to see how issues of professionalism and commercialism are addressed in the area of licensing for physicians. Finally, we will examine the actual adjudication practices of one state board.

TWO EXAMPLES OF COMMERCIALISM

Case Example #1: Physicians and the Rise of the Contract Research Industry

Clinical medical research is a multibillion-dollar corporate enterprise in the United States today.[4] At any one time, there are over twenty-five hundred Food and Drug Administration (FDA)–approved clinical trials taking place in this country, in addition to non-FDA and other types of clinical trials taking place in the United States and abroad. All these trials require patients/subjects, sometimes in the thousands, and acquiring these patients/subjects is the single most difficult (and expensive) aspect of any clinical trial.[5] Academic health centers, the traditional "home" of most drug trials (which is no longer the case), do not have access to the number, type, and range of patients needed for all these trials. This lack of capacity has created a new for-profit industry—contract research organizations (CROs)—to meet these clinical research needs.[6] A relative organizational nonentity a decade ago, over a thousand private for-profit CROs providing a range of services to the medical research industry now exist. These services range from specific subcontract work (e.g., statistical analysis or recruiting and providing research subjects) to more "full-service" needs such as developing actual project designs, supervising data collection or data analysis, generating study reports, and even authoring the articles that will appear in the scientific literature.[7] Clinical research has become a "big business." Several of these companies trade on the New York and related stock exchanges.[8] Many of the CROs that operate today were founded by physicians, academics, and former pharmaceutical industry employees.[9]

Of all the services provided by CROs, perhaps the most difficult (and therefore the most lucrative) is securing the necessary number and types of patients for trials.[10] Challenges include finding enough patients of a particular (and vulnerable) social group (e.g., children)[11] or adults with specific disease patterns (e.g., a group of women with severe rheumatoid arthritis). One strategy adopted by CROs is to compile (and market) a proprietary database of potential subjects, organized by demographic and disease profiles.[12] Another approach is to establish a nationwide web of community physicians who will be responsible for identifying among their own patients appropriate research subjects. In this latter example, the referring physician can be compensated anywhere from $1,500 for "routine" patients to as much as $40,000 for patients with rare conditions. Rather than pay the physician directly for his or her referral with what amounts to a "finder's fee," a customary arrangement is for the enrolling physician to collect the necessary blood or tissue samples from the patient and then for the CRO to reimburse the doctor for "clinical research services." Such reimbursements, however, are considerably larger than the usual reimbursement received for running the same tests for regular patients not enrolled in research studies. Other reimbursement schemes include paying the referring physician for "consultation" on the underlying research project, or engaging him or her as a speaker to tout research results. Particularly active referring physicians may even have their names included on research publications, which may themselves be ghost written by the sponsoring company or organization.[13] Top physician recruiters of patients for clinical research can earn between five hundred thousand and one million dollars per year over and above their regular practice income.[14]

Case Example #2: Physicians and the Sale of Consumer Products

A second example of commercialism we will draw upon in this chapter is the sale of health- and nonhealth-related products by physicians to their patients and/or the public at large. Examples range from selling such products out of one's office to hawking products via television advertising, infomercials, and the Internet. An illustrative example is the $26 billion skin care industry.[15] One of the newer marketing ploys is the sale of "physician-developed" preparations such as anti-aging formulas, "cosmeceutical" creams, or "skin doctors' dermaceuticals." Often these products are available only through an office visit replete with a consulting fee charge. A few of the more entrepreneurial physicians have achieved celebrity status with frequent television appearances, publicity campaigns, and book signings.[16] Although terms such as "cosmeceutical" are not staples within academic medical circles, they are extremely lucrative identifiers within the skin care industry.

There is, however, a more important story than the admittedly limited one of medicine and cosmetics. In 1997, the *Wall Street Journal* published a front-page story on physicians as product distributors: "First Do No Harm: Second, Peddle a Box of All Fabric Bleach—Doctors Upset Over Lower Pay are Selling Amway Products: Not Everyone Gets Rich."[17] The resulting firestorm brought a swift—although controversial and eventually muddled—response from organized medicine. One of the first responses was from the AMA Council on Ethical and Judicial Affairs, which issued an opinion recommending restrictions on the sale of health- and nonhealth-related products from physician offices. Then, in November 1997, the AMA weekly newspaper, *AMNews*, published an overview of the controversy, with the startling revelation that "tens of thousands" of physicians had joined the ranks of "network marketers."[18] In December of that year, the AMA House of Delegates debated restricting the sale of health- and nonhealth-related products by doctors. Particular constituencies (e.g., dermatology and plastic surgery) were vociferous in protesting any regulatory intrusions over what were, for them, longstanding commercial practices. Reflecting the debate (and underlying schisms), the opinion eventually adopted by the Council on Ethical and Judicial Affairs targeted only nonhealth-related products. A year and a half later, at the June 1999 annual meeting and amidst continued controversy and rounds of modifications, the final opinion approved by the AMA was a compromise that pleased few. According to one delegate they were "broad guidelines, not commandments, that give doctors room to wiggle."[19]

Meanwhile, ever-new issues of physician commercialism continued to assault the public during the two years (1997–1999) of AMA debate.[20] Not to be undone by the entrepreneurial excesses of its members, the AMA announced in August 1997 that it had entered into a product-endorsement relationship with Sunbeam.[21] Medical leaders such as Arnold Relman, Jerome Kassirer, and George Lundberg were aghast.[22] Although the AMA would quickly recant, the damage had been done. Organized medicine, it appeared to many, had "sold out to big business."

THE CODES OF PROFESSIONAL BEHAVIOR AND THEIR RESPONSE TO COMMERCIALISM

The AMA *Principles of Medical Ethics*

The most recent version of the AMA *Principles of Medical Ethics* was adopted by the AMA House of Delegates in 2001.[23] Issues of commercialism are not mentioned in this document. The closest possible link to the dangers of commercialism directs physicians to "uphold the standards of professionalism, [and to] be honest in all professional interactions."

Considering our case studies, the charge to physicians that they be honest in their professional interactions appears straightforward. Telling a patient that he or she is undergoing "treatment" when the patient is actually a research subject would certainly violate this tenet. Failing to inform the patient, even in the absence of a direct question, also would violate this principle. But the sale of products is more nebulous. Telling a patient, directly or indirectly, that he or she needs a health- or nonhealth-related product might be untruthful in some cases. Similarly, commercial behaviors of this type might be considered a failure to "uphold the standards of professionalism." There is, however, no specific language in *Principles* that prohibits commercial activities or even suggests that some types of commercialism might be ethically inappropriate. Furthermore, there is no specific language in *Principles* prohibiting conflicts of interest, a general category of behaviors frequently associated with commercial activities. Finally, and given all the media attention and ethical concerns that circulated in the late 1990s about AMA and physician commercialism, it is indeed odd that the 2001 edition of *Principles* fails to mention commercialism in any form or fashion. It's not that organized medicine has lacked the opportunity. The 2001 *Principles* replaced a document that had been last changed in 1990, and there are extensive differences between the two editions—just not with respect to medical commercialism.

The AMA *Declaration of Professional Responsibility*

The AMA *Declaration of Professional Responsibility: Medicine's Social Contract with Humanity* was passed in 2001 by the AMA House of Delegates.[24] It is an oath reflecting the challenges facing twenty-first-century physicians and written for "the world community of physicians." The *Declaration's* preamble addresses contemporary threats to medicine's professionalism, but the document itself gives only passing attention to issues of commercialism. In the third part of the *Declaration*, physicians are urged "to treat the sick and injured with competence and compassion and without prejudice" while *Declaration VI* declares, "Work freely with colleagues to discover, develop, and promote advances in medicine and public health that ameliorate suffering and contribute to human well-being." It would be a stretch to argue that "without prejudice" refers to a patient's ability to pay, or that *Declaration VI*'s command to "work freely" implies that physicians should work sans financial remuneration. More likely, the call to work freely calls upon physicians to resist limitations on the free exchange of scientific knowledge in light of the numerous and widely reported restrictions placed by industry on the publication of industry-sponsored research findings.[25] This is, however, as close as we come to issues of commercialism within the *Declaration*. Of related interest, the only time we see the term "professionalism" is in the title of the *Declaration* and in its last line: "We make these promises solemnly, freely, and upon our personal and professional honor."

The AMA *Current Opinions with Annotations*

The AMA 2004 *Code of Medical Ethics: Current Opinions with Annotations (O&A)* is the most comprehensive of the six documents reviewed in this chapter.[26] References to commercialism are scattered throughout *O&A*. These a reference to "health care facility ownership by a physician," material about "gifts to physicians from industry," and specific comments about the sale of health and nonhealth-related goods from physicians' offices and/or Web sites.

For example, opinion E-8.062 (nonhealth-related goods) certainly appears unequivocal in rejecting physician sales: "Physicians should not sell nonhealth-related goods from their offices or other treatment setting." The opinion specifies that such practices are a conflict of interest for physicians, and that they "threaten to erode the primary obligation of physicians to serve the interests of their patients before their own," and "risk demeaning the practice of medicine." This ban, however, comes with its own list of exceptions and exemptions. For example, E-8.062 states that exceptions are allowed if the goods benefit community organizations, if they are "low-cost," if physicians "take no share in profit from their sale," if the goods are not a regular part of the physician's business, if the transaction is "conducted in a dignified manner," and if physicians do not pressure patients.

Stipulations concerning the sale of health-related products (E-8.063) are more detailed and include references to several other opinions.[27] In E-8.063, the sale of health-related products is framed as a "conflict of interest," a practice that "threatens to erode patient trust," and one that undermines the primary obligation of physicians to "serve the interests of their patients before their own." Like opinion E-8.062 (nonhealth-related goods), E-8.063 also lists exceptions and conditions under which the sale of health products may take place, including the sale of those products that "serve the immediate and pressing needs of patients," where access to the product would be limited (e.g., because of rural location), and when no profit is made. Other restrictions specify that physicians must disclose information regarding financial arrangements with the manufacturer or supplier, and a prohibition against physician participation in "exclusive distributorships," a ban that has particular relevance to some of the cosmetic sales mentioned above.

The *O&A* contains specifics about our second case example, physician behavior in clinical research. Examples include subject selection for clinical trials, commercial use of human tissue, conflicts of interest in biomedical research, and the management of conflicts in the conduct of clinical trials. The opening sentence of the section on "Managing Conflicts" (section E-8.0315) is worth citing because of how it captures a number of dimensions regarding physician commercialism: "Avoidance of real or perceived conflicts of interest in clinical research is imperative if the medical community is to ensure objectivity and maintain individual and institutional integrity."[28] Physician compensation is specifically discussed, and there is specific language prohibiting the inappropriately high remuneration paid to physicians by CROs for taking vital signs or other relatively minor examinations or procedures ("any remuneration received by the researcher from the company whose product is being studied must be commensurate with the efforts of the researcher on behalf of the company").

In sum, *O&A* contains language that specifically covers our two case examples. It also speaks to other public scandals involving inappropriate commercial behaviors of physicians. The key issue here—and in all six documents covered in this chapter—is whether physicians are subject to peer review on the basis of these standards. As we will discuss below, the answers are not that clear or forthcoming.

American College of Physicians' *Ethics Manual* (Fourth Edition)

In terms of size and specificity, the American College of Physicians (ACP) *Ethics Manual*[29] falls somewhere between the shorter AMA *Principles of Medical Ethics* and the highly detailed AMA *Opinions with Annotations.* Although the *Manual* does address patient interests, the language used is not uniformly clear as to whose interests should prevail. In the section on "The Changing Practice Environment," the *Manual* states 1) "Physicians must promote their patients' welfare in an increasingly complex health care system," 2) "The physician must seek to ensure that the medically appropriate level of care takes primacy over financial considerations imposed by the physician's own practice, investments, or financial arrangements," and 3) "although the physician should be fairly compensated for services rendered, a sense of duty to the patient should take precedence over concern about compensation when a patient's well-being is at stake." While the terminology appears unambiguous in the case of a critically ill patient with no money, for example, it is awash with ambiguity when the patient's health status is not so critical.

Material on financial conflicts also is confusing. The *Manual* is the only one of the six documents reviewed that specifically acknowledges that there is research on the impact of gifts on clinical decision making ("the acceptance of even small gifts has been documented to affect clinical judgment and heightens the perception [as well as the reality] of a conflict of interest").[30] The *Manual* also specifies that the appearance of financial influence may be just as damaging as actual malfeasance. Nonetheless, when it comes to actually accepting gifts, trips, and the like, these practices are only "strongly discouraged" rather than being prohibited. Furthermore, the *Manual* enjoins physicians to "critically evaluate medical information provided by detail persons, advertisements, or industry-sponsored educational programs," even as it informs readers that there is research establishing that physicians can be notoriously poor judges of what does and does not influence their clinical decision making.[31] In short, while the *Manual* reminds readers in several places that the patient's welfare and best interests must be the prime consideration, the *Manual* remains internally inconsistent around specific do's and don'ts.

Finally, like all documents that detail professional standards, the *Manual* contains instances of what might be labeled "ethical smoke and mirrors." For example, while the *Manual* specifically mentions paying physicians to provide research subjects, it does so with language that condemns only the payment of finder's fees ("giving finder's fees to individual physicians for referring patients to a research project generates an unethical conflict of interest"). The *Manual*, however, ignores the payments to physicians under the guise of "consultation" and "research" when the amount of reimbursement paid for work on behalf of CRO is far in excess of what anyone might consider (except, it seems, the CRO and physician) usual and customary.

The Federation of State Medical Boards' *A Guide to the Essentials of Modern Medical Practice* (Tenth edition): "Disciplinary Action against Licensees: Grounds for Action"

The Federation of State Medical Boards is the professional association for seventy medical boards in the United States and its territories. Among other functions, it publishes *A Guide to the Essentials of Modern Medical Practice Act*.[32] The *Essentials* contains a suggested forty-three principles that state medical boards can use in drawing up their own set of standards of professional behavior. While the actual standards employed by individual states can differ in both context and content, most rely heavily on the *Essentials,* and thus this document serves as a guide to what may be considered "unprofessional or dishonorable conduct." The *Essentials* contains a set of unprofessional behaviors and their possible commercial implications. These standards would seem to cover some of the examples of recruiting patients for CROs or taking advantage in selling products to patients.

If the *Essentials* is viewed as a master list of professional values with disciplinary implications, and if we are to better understand the relation of unprincipled commercialism to professional behaviors, then three questions must be addressed. First, in a broad sense, how do the standards of particular state codes mirror the overall range of behaviors captured in the *Essentials*? For example, what items are contained in a state code, and what ends up being omitted? Second, now that we know what is different (what was left out, what was added), how are the various grounds for discipline actually worded? What modifiers (e.g., verbs, adjectives, and adverbs) are used to give a particular emphasis or spin to a given item in the code? Third, and perhaps most

Table 4.1. Unprofessional Behaviors with Possible Commercial Implications as Specified in the *Guide to the Essentials of Modern Medical Practice Act*

Standard #	Type of Behavior
4	"conduct likely to deceive, defraud or harm the public"
6	"making a false or misleading statement regarding his or her skill or the efficacy or value of" treatments prescribed
7	representing that an incurable condition, sickness, disease or injury can be cured
9	"negligence in the practice of medicine as determined by the Board"
23	"obtaining any fee by fraud, deceit or misrepresentation"
25	being paid for services not rendered with exceptions for legal partnerships, etc.
36	conduct that brings "the medical profession into disrepute, including but not limited to violation of any provision of a national code of ethics acknowledged by the Board"
40	"conduct that violates patient trust and exploits the physician-patient relationship for personal gain"
41	failure-to-act provisions, including: failure to provide appropriate care, to refer, or to protest "inappropriate managed care denials" when "such actions are taken for the sole purpose of positively influencing the physician's or the plan's financial well being"

important, how are items that pertain to inappropriate commercial behavior actually enforced?

This third question will be addressed farther on. If we return to our case examples for just a minute, although specific issues such as patient recruitment into clinical trials are not mentioned in the *Essentials*, the general standards seem sufficiently robust to address the concerns raised in this chapter. The rub, as always, is how state boards actually interpret and apply their code in the regulation of physician practice behaviors.

Medical Professionalism in the New Millennium: A Physician Charter

The *Charter* is a collaborative effort of organizations for specialists in internal medicine in the United States and Europe.[33] Of the six documents reviewed here, it is the only one that explicitly acknowledges the deleterious influence of market forces, the temptations of self-interest, and the need to subjugate self-interest to patient well-being. The preamble unequivocally states that professionalism is "the basis of medicine's contract with society" and that professionalism "demands placing the interests of patients above those of the physician." Conflicts of interest are specifically addressed. Physicians are reminded that there are "many opportunities to compromise their professional responsibilities by pursuing private gain or personal advantage." Moreover, readers are told that these compromises are "especially threatening in the pursuit of personal or organizational interactions with for-profit industries, including medical equipment manufacturers, insurance companies, and pharmaceutical firms." The *Charter* contains several explicit references to "market forces," such as the observation that market forces are a threat to medical professionalism and the primacy of patient welfare, and that "increasing dependence on market forces to transform health care systems, and the temptations for physicians to forsake their traditional commitment to the primacy of patients' interests" weakens the "fidelity of medicine's social contract during this turbulent time."[34]

The *Charter* represents an optimal balance between the broadly framed and ethereally worded *Principles* and the mind-numbing density of *O&A*. Furthermore, the *Charter* is unique in identifying self and peer review as essential to professionalism. On a negative note, the *Charter* does not acknowledge, as does the ACP *Manual*, that there is research demonstrating how medical marketing and research practices affect physicians' decision making. Unfortunately, there is no single document that merges the *Charter*'s emphasis on self-review with the ACP *Manual* recognition that physicians are prone to considerable self-deception in thinking that they are above the fray and are not, like their peers, influenced by commercial pressures. Whether driven by hubris or innocence, the weakest link in medicine's chain of professionalism is the tendency to acknowledge the impact of medical commercialism on peers, but not on oneself.

In summary, of the six documents reviewed, on issues of commercialism and professionalism the *Charter* best speaks to medical students, residents, and practicing clinicians across the spectrum of medical education and clinical practice.

THE LITERATURE ON STATE BOARD
ACTIONS AND COMMERCIALISM

When Physicians Go Wrong: Commercialism and
State Boards of Medical Examiners

No single aspect of medical professionalism has been so consistently criticized, both internally and externally, as the unwillingness and/or inability of organized medicine to regulate itself in the public's interest. [35] Nonetheless, the issue has received little coverage within the medical literature. An examination of the *Annals of Internal Medicine*, the *Journal of the American Medical Association* (*JAMA*), and the *New England Journal of Medicine* finds that only *JAMA* has devoted even a modicum of editorial and research coverage to this issue.[36] Even here, the bulk of *JAMA*'s most recent coverage appears in a single, and now somewhat dated (1998) calendar year.

Taken as a whole, the studies that have been published illustrate why we know so little about physician disciplinary proceedings. First, most studies of physician discipline are state specific (e.g., California, Ohio). Second, most physician-discipline studies focus on a specific type of transgression—the two most common are "impairment due to drugs or alcohol"[37] and "disciplines due to sex and/or inappropriate patient contact."[38] Third—and a point we will revisit—different states report vastly different discipline rates for the same types of offenses, suggesting the possibility of significant variability in how different state boards interpret the same kind of statutes. For example, in two studies that employed the same study methodology, 34 percent of the physicians disciplined in California were convicted of "negligence or incompetence" versus only 7 percent in Ohio.[39] Conversely, Ohio's major conviction category was "impairment due to alcohol and/or drug use" at 21 percent versus California's rate of 12 percent.

There are fifty state medical boards (not including that of the District of Columbia), each with its own set of physician misconduct standards and each with its own way of doing business. Moreover, most boards function in relative obscurity. When media coverage does appear, usually it is critical. Examples include Sidney Wolfe's *New York Times* editorial, "Bad Doctors Get a Free Ride," Robert Pear's *New York Times* article "Inept Physicians are Rarely Listed as Law Requires," *USA Today* editorial "HMOs Give Bad Doctors a Pass, Put Patients at Risk: 84% Reported Nothing to National Databank in Past Decade," and Christopher Gearon's AARP online piece, "Unmasking Unsafe Doctors."[40] On a more positive note, articles about unprofessional physician behavior often urge readers to become more proactive with respect to their own health care and check either their state medical board or a national resource (such as the Federation of State Medical Boards' "DocInfo" database) to see whether their physician has had actions taken against, or restrictions placed on, his or her license.[41]

Although media coverage of state board actions is infrequent, there is one pattern of media coverage worth noting. Public Citizen's Health Research Group (HRG) is the most aggressive watchdog of state board actions and publishes a variety of reports on state board activities.[42] Examples include a "Survey of Doctor Disciplinary Information on State Medical Board Web

Sites" (HRG 1506) and "Ranking of State Medical Board Serious Disciplinary Actions in 2003" (HRG 1696). When media articles do appear, they tend to be ignited by Public Citizen's release of its annual state rankings. The typical pattern is for an initial wave of national coverage (e.g., the *New York Times, USA Today*) followed by a secondary wave of state-focused coverage, that coverage being positive or negative in tone depending on the state's ranking. Examples include *Business Journal's* ranking of Minnesota as "one of the worst states in the country at policing its doctors," (and a ranking as forty-fourth in the nation in health care in 2002), and its assessments of Florida ("Medical Board Still Falls Short in Doc Discipline," or "Low Ratings a Bitter Pill for Medical Board") versus those of Missouri and Kansas ("Missouri, Kansas Rank Well for Disciplinary Actions against Doctors").[43]

The Web Sites of Five State Medical Boards

Examining the websites of state boards to ascertain the type and frequency of physician offenses is a frustrating undertaking.[44] While all state boards have a Web site, not all boards post physician offense data. Furthermore, when states do post data, not all present that data in a way that allows visitors to compile aggregate information on types of violations and prevalence. As an unsystematic experiment, I visited the websites of the first five states, in alphabetical order (Alabama, Alaska, Arizona, Arkansas, and California).[45]

The Alabama State Board of Medical Examiner's website contains a link to "Public Disciplinary Actions," but the information provided, which includes determination, physician name, action taken, license number, and town address, does not include information on actual offenses.

The home page of the Alaska State Medical Board does present the underlying cause for board actions, but in a rather strange (incomplete) manner.[46] The board's website contains no data or links to data. Instead there are links to two isolated newsletters for "summer 2001" and "spring 2002." Both contain information on physician offenses. The spring 2002 newsletter, for example, contains information on board actions that includes the physician's name, decision date, and decision (e.g., "reprimand, Civil Fine of $3,500 with $1,500 Suspended") as well as the reason for the decision ("allegation that respondent may be unsafe to practice due to personal health concerns; allegation of history of medication abuse"). Nonetheless, the two newsletters are the extent of Alaska's disclosure.

The home page of the Arizona State Medical Board contains a link to "Recent Actions" (located under the primary link "Consumer Center").[47] The list covers board actions for the past twenty-four months with data including the physician's name, medical number, licensee city, and a description of the action. Examples of the descriptions include the cryptic "Decree of Censure for failure to return to the hosp to prop eval the stability for trnsfr of pt, failure to return to hosp in timely manner when pt in post-op shock, failure to eval pt in labor for 12 hrs. Prob until completion of 20 hrs CME. See Order." In addition there is a PDF link labeled "View Full Documentation," which contains the file of record for the action and the complete findings of fact. In short, Arizona's data is voluminous and essentially complete.

The home page for the Arkansas State Medical Board contains two links that might be of relevance, a "Data Portal" and "Information."[48] The "Data Portal" service is described on the Web site as "currently unavailable" and has been so for well over a year.[49] The "Information" link provides access to "board notices, a listing of" actions of the board back to January 1, 2003, and an "online newsletter." Both the notices and newsletter contain exactly the same data regarding physician disciplinary action, including the name, license number, action of the board, date of the action, and town address of the physician.

Finally, the home page for the California Board of Medical Examiners contains no direct links to information about state board actions.[50] Instead, viewers are provided with a list of information that is available (e.g., accusation, decision, and the stipulated agreement) as well as a list of information that is not available (e.g., complaints, pending malpractice cases). In turn, viewers must submit the name of a specific physician, and if an "enforcement" (to use the California board's terminology) has taken place or is pending, the details of this enforcement are provided only when one completes the required form, mails or faxes it to the board, and pays the required document fee.

Nationally, the Federation of State Medical Boards' annual *Summary of Board Actions* provides detailed data on sanctions applied by all state boards, but nothing on the type of offense.[51] Public Citizen does provide data on the types of offenses on a state-by-state basis. Public Citizen groups its data into seven headings: 1) "criminal conviction;" 2) "sexual abuse or sexual misconduct with a patient;" 3) "substandard care, incompetence or negligence;" 4) "overprescribing or misprescribing drugs;" 5) "substance abuse;" 6) "disciplinary action by another state or agency;" and 7) "other offenses."[52] None of these headings explicitly addresses issues of commercialism.

Public Citizen does, however, provide a list of thirty-seven different examples of unprofessional behavior that it defines as more serious than "professional misconduct," but that does not fit into the seven categories listed previously. Several of these thirty-seven examples appear to be related to commercial issues. These include: "selling drugs and devices for financial gain," "fraud in medical research," "ordering or performing unnecessary or inappropriate procedure for a patient deliberately, rather than because of incompetence," and "accepting payments from laboratories for sending patients' tests." The list also identifies violations under the category "failure to comply with a professional rule." Examples associated with this category of noncompliance include: "violation of restrictions on advertising," "requiring patients to purchase drugs or devices from a physician," "employing an agent to solicit patients," "endorsing a product," "fee-splitting," "two-tiered billing," and "non-payment of student loan." What is not clear is whether data relevant to these additional types of unprofessional commercialism are available from Public Citizen. As noted previously, the only data it publishes are grouped by the seven categories listed in the preceding paragraph, and these categories do not discriminate for commercial activities.

Finally, Public Citizen maintains an "interactive database" which offers a state-by-state checklist of the kinds of information (e.g., "Action Taken," "Offense," "Board Orders") provided by the fifty state boards and the board of the District of Columbia. There is, however, no information that allows determination of what boards might consider to be unprofessional commercialism.

In summary, data on unprofessional commercial behavior by physicians are hard to come by, and this includes data from published studies, national databases, or state board Web sites. Of the five state boards reviewed, even when data were provided (Alaska and Arizona) there were no examples of physician commercial misconduct. In other words, while at least some state boards appear to have the statutory regulatory tools, there is little or no indication that unprofessional commercial actions by physicians are of particular concern to these boards.

A Case Example: One State Board

The state board that is reviewed here does have regulations that explicitly cover unprofessional commercial behaviors. The state prohibits "conduct likely to deceive, defraud, or harm the public," "fee splitting," "abusive or fraudulent billing," and "referral to another provider or facility in which the physician has a "financial or economic interest," as well as two examples that are particularly relevant to this chapter: 1) "paying, offering to pay, receiving, or agreeing to receive a commission, rebate, or remuneration, directly or indirectly, primarily for the referral of patients of the prescription of drugs or devices," and 2) "dispensing for any profit any drug or device, unless the physician has disclosed the physician's own profit interest."

This state medical board has the statutory ability to handle our two case examples (listed in the previous section of this chapter), as well as a range of other violations of professional commercialism. What we do not know at this point is whether this board actively seeks out and prosecutes occurrences of unprofessional commercialism. I used two routes to answer this question.

The first approach was to visit the state's Web site as outlined above for the five state boards. This search revealed that this state board does provide online data about unprofessional behaviors, but only in a limited fashion and for a short time period (eight months). Examples of published offenses were for sex with patients, substance abuse, and improper prescribing. There was no mention of discipline for unprofessional commercialism.

The second approach was a series of interviews conducted with past and present physician members of this board and with state board officials. The interviews focused on issues of commercialism in medicine. One overall finding was that this board operates under a normative framework with respect to how members view their responsibilities (it's "how we do things around here"). One individual described the board's role as: "protecting the public rather than enforcing medical ethics." Other members noted that there must be a "clear and compelling danger" to the public or to an individual before the board acts. For example, this state board considers itself to be aggressive in prosecuting physicians who have sexually assaulted patients or who were impaired due to drug or alcohol abuse. However, members would not be inclined to act in the hypothetical case of a drug company making payments to physicians to prescribe their drug instead of a competitor's (the interview question specified that both drugs were FDA approved and appropriate for the condition for which the practitioner is prescribing). Nor was there any likelihood of action (per a specific interview question) for physicians who were paid to give talks to peers supporting the off-label use of a drug. In the words of one board member, "At best, [the physician] would receive a mild hand slap." Further questions and board members' answers made it compellingly clear that this board is not inclined to act when the issue is internal to the profession of medicine (actions or behaviors between or among physicians) even though such issues would reflect on the integrity of the profession or its perceived trustworthiness.

A second insight is that while board members were willing to agree (in principle) with some of the professional commercialism standards contained in some of the documents we reviewed earlier (e.g., the AMA *O&A* or the Federation's *Essentials*) they did not consider these standards as grounds for board action. Even violations of the board's regulations concerning commercial malfeasance were not to be pursued unless public safety was at stake. In short, what the board actually prosecutes is a subset of its own statutes.

A third insight is that boards face structural limitations with respect to which violations to enforce and discipline. During their interviews, board members discussed the "limited resources" available, the need to "pick out cases" and the resulting approach of being "more reactive than proactive." Because of limited resources, the public or another physician must file a complaint with the board before the board will move. Thus, this board, in all likelihood, would not act against a physician if an organization (e.g., hospital, clinic, chain) were found guilty of commercial malfeasance, even if it was a physician who carried out the behavior for which the company was convicted. The one exception that was noted in the interviews was if a physician were convicted of fraud in state or federal court. Here, the board might revoke or suspend the license of the physician if he or she were found guilty of criminal behavior (grounds found in almost all state codes).

In summary, even though a state board might have the statutory tools to target unprofessional commercialism, there are a number of factors, structural and normative, that can redirect or limit the attention paid to improper commercial activity.

A PROPOSED SOLUTION

Even though the particulars reported previously may not be surprising to some, it is rather disconcerting to find such a large gap between organized medicine's denunciation of physician commercialism and the relative lack of attention paid to commercialism at the level of peer review. At the same time, we now know that some states already have regulations in place that can address the behaviors outlined in our case examples as well as other kinds of unprofessional commercialism.

While it might be easy to point to all this dissonance and demand that medicine enforce its own rules, it is not exactly clear whether a simple "just say no" (to unprofessional commercial behaviors) would solve the situation. Exactly how are we supposed to encourage physicians to adopt a lower commercial profile while organizations and health-care systems continue to operate within an overall capitalist system? An outright ban on all types of commercial behavior by physicians most certainly would be naive as well as counterproductive, unenforceable, and perhaps even ethically problematic. Similar calls to tighten up enforcement and punishment for unprofessional commercialism, while having some appeal to this writer (after all, actions do speak louder than words) may provoke resistance from organized medicine's internal membership.

What I wish to propose, then, is a series of action steps. These steps would require organized medicine to become more aggressive and proactive with regard to physician commercial behaviors. At the same time, these steps would (hopefully) undercut the possibility that peers would simply abandon self-regulation or flee to some sort of commercial underground to continue their activities. While the devil is always in the details, the core of this proposal is the use of existing prohibitions against commercialism (our unnamed state board described previously could serve as an example) to enforce aggressively those standards, and to cite violations in detail and for the record—but with punishment being the publication of all findings of fault. In other words, while there would be aggressive and comprehensive determining of facts, there would be no suspensions, no revocations of licenses, and no remedial classes. Instead, the plan (and hope) is that the absence of traditional sanctions will promote a more aggressive state board action at the evidentiary stage of peer review.

Physicians who sell soap powders, for example, must face a regulatory board of their peers and explain and defend their actions. The first layer of sanctions, therefore, is the peer-review process itself. When fault is found, board findings must be for the record, and all specifics must be listed. These determinations would then be made part of the public record, including online accessibility, and perhaps even posted in the offending physician's offices.

The other side of the regulatory coin focuses on physicians. They can be as commercial as they wish, and do so without the threat of having their licenses revoked or of having to attend mandatory rehabilitative class. The state and/ or federal court system would still target things such as Medicare fraud, but these findings of guilt and punitive consequences would not (necessarily) result in the loss of one's license. What the physician risks is another citation and another line on his or her disciplinary record. The public can decide whether or not to seek treatment from a physician with such citations.

The key here is to remember that this process of adjudication and findings of fault are specific to issues of unprofessional commercialism. Physicians who rape a patient or deal drugs to minors would still be subject to the traditional system. The changes proposed here are specific to issues of unprofessional commercialism and allow the public to see that organized medicine is serious and committed when it describes certain types of commercial behavior as unprofessional. It also allows the public to make final decisions about seeking the services of physicians who are cited. This provides a kind of market-based solution to a market-based problem. The two bumps in the road are the willingness of organized medicine to take such a step and whether the public cares enough to work with the provided information.

CONCLUSIONS

In this chapter, we examined the relationship between medicine as a profession and medicine as an object of commerce. We opened with an overview of organized medicine's public denouncement of commercialism during the 1980s and 1990s. We then examined six statements of professional ethics/ principles to see how issues of "unprofessional commercialism" were addressed. We then explored how state boards of medical examiners confront—both in statute and in practice—physician commercial behaviors. Our operational thesis throughout was as follows: "if organized medicine truly believes commercialism to be antithetical to core professional values, then we should see evidence of this concern within the work of medical boundary setting—be that in core statements of professional values and/or in the work of peer review.

Overall, we encountered a decidedly equivocal picture. Some professional statements contain clear warnings about commercialism, while others speak volumes by remaining mute on the subject. Some state boards have adopted statutory tools to address physician commercialism, while others either had not used or do not use the tools they have. When we examined the practices of one state medical board, we found that this body had created a set of working principles inconsistent with its own statutory rules. Board members and administrators drew an explicit line between "protecting the public" and what it viewed (in a lesser sense) as "enforcing medical ethics." In short, this board's biggest impediment in dealing with issues of commercialism proved to be normative rather than statutory. Despite specific rules that actual injury to patients "need not be established," the board chose to direct its energies toward cases involving actual injury or harm to patients and thus further marginalized issues of economic damage. When it came to censuring unprofessional behavior, this board preferred that commercial violations (e.g., fraud) be "preadjudicated" in state or federal court. Finally, members of the board drew clear distinctions between physician behaviors that are clearly illegal (e.g., Medicare fraud) and those that are, in the words of one board member, "just unprofessional," and in the words of another, "merely distasteful."

Issues of commercialism will continue to plague organized medicine because of such renderings. Organized medicine has undertaken a number of efforts, particularly within medical education, to refocus and reenergize medical professionalism.[53] These efforts are both substantive and laudatory. Nonetheless, if organized medicine is not willing to narrow the gap between rhetoric and reality and, in particular, between the classroom and the clinic, then all the codes and charters will be for naught. No one advocates teaching one standard of evidence-based medicine in the classroom and then practicing another in the clinic. Professionalism should be held to the same benchmark.

In the end, actions do speak louder than words. For this reason we have focused on actions, or the products of actions, in this chapter. Organized medicine may continue to denounce commercialism, but unless it is willing to directly confront the unprofessional commercial behaviors of its members, and until it is willing to forego its traditional rationalizations against action, then organized medicine will continue to perpetuate a rhetoric that will ultimately contribute to its own demise.

NOTES

1. M. Angell, "Is Academic Medicine for Sale?" *New England Journal of Medicine* 342 (2000): 1516–18; M. Angell, "The Pharmaceutical Industry: To Whom Is It Accountable?" *New England Journal of Medicine* 342 (2000): 1902–4; M. Angell, *The Truth about the Drug Companies: How They Deceive Us and What To Do about It* (New York: Random House, 2004); J. A. Barondess, "Medicine and Professionalism," *Archives of Internal Medicine* 163 (2003): 145–49; G. D. Lundberg, "Medicine: A Profession in Trouble?" *Journal of the American Medical Association* 253 (1985): 2879–80; G. D. Lundberg, "Countdown to Millennium: Balancing the Professionalism and Business of Medicine: Medicine's Rocking Horse," *Journal of the American Medical Association* 263 (1990): 86–87; G. D. Lundberg, "Promoting Professionalism through Self-Appraisal in this Critical Decade," *Journal of the American Medical Association* 265 (1991): 2859; G. D. Lundberg, "A Pendulum Swings and a Rocking Horse Rocks," *Journal of the American Medical Association* 278 (1997):1703–4; G. D. Lundberg, *Severed Trust: Why American Medicine Can't Be Fixed* (New York: Basic Books, 2001); J. P. Kassirer, "Academic Medical Centers Under Siege," *New England Journal of Medicine* 331 (1994): 1370–71; J. P. Kassirer, "Managed Care and the Morality of the Marketplace," *New England Journal of Medicine* 333 (1995): 50–52; J. P. Kassirer, "Our Endangered Integrity: It Can Only Get Worse," *New England Journal of Medicine* 336 (1997): 1666–67; J. P. Kassirer, "Managing Managed Care's Tarnished Image," *New England Journal of Medicine* 337 (1997): 338–39; J. P. Kassirer, "Managing Care—Should We Adopt a New Ethic?" *New England Journal of Medicine* 339 (1998): 397–98; J. P. Kassirer, *On the Take: How Medicine's Complicity with Big Business Can Endanger Your Health* (New York: Oxford University Press, 2004); J. H. McArthur and F. D. Moore, "The Two Cultures and the Health Care Revolution," *Journal of the American Medical Association* 277 (1997): 985–89; F. Mullan and G. Lundberg, "Looking Back, Looking Forward: Straight Talk about U.S. Medicine," 2000, 80-weblinks1.epnet.com.floyd.lib.umn.edu/citation.asp?tb = 1&_ua = bo + B%5F + shn + 1 + db + aphjnh + bt + ID + + HAF + 4FBB&_ug = sid + 0FFE5C17% 2D215D%2D4650%2DA86F%2D40A82E4A7DF0%40sessionmgr2 + dbs + aph + 650 A&_us = hd + False + fcl + Aut + or + Date + frn + 1 + sm + KS + sl + %2D1 + dstb + KS + ri + KAAACBZD00023458 + 5688&_uh = btn + N + 6C9C&_uso = st%5B0 + %2DJN + + %22Health + + Affairs%22 + + and + + DT + + 20000101 + tg%5B0 + %2D + db%

5B0 + %2Daph + hd + False + op%5B0 + %2D + mdb%5B0 + %2Dimh + 9F30&fn = 1&r
n = 7 (accessed August 4, 2005); E. D. Pellegrino and A. S. Relman, "Professional Medical Associations: Ethical and Practical Guidelines," *Journal of the American Medical Association* 282 (1999): 984–86; A. S. Relman, "The New Medical-Industrial Complex," *New England Journal of Medicine* 303 (1980): 963–70; A. S. Relman, "Practicing Medicine in the New Business Climate," *New England Journal of Medicine* 316 (1987): 1150–51; A. S. Relman, "Shattuck Lecture: The Health Care Industry: Where Is It Taking Us?" *New England Journal of Medicine* 325 (1991): 854–59; A. S. Relman, "What Market Values Are Doing to Medicine," *National Forum* 73 (1993): 17–21; A. S. Relman, "Medical Practice under the Clinton Reforms: Avoiding Domination by Business," *New England Journal of Medicine* 329 (1993): 1574–76; A. S. Relman, "Dr. Business," *American Prospect* 8 (1997): 91–95; A. S. Relman, "Education to Defend Professional Values in the New Corporate Age," *Academic Medicine* 73 (1998): 1229–33; A. S. Relman and M. Angell, "America's Other Drug Problem: How the Drug Industry Distorts Medicine and Politics," *New Republic*, December 16, 2002, S27–S41; A. S. Relman and G. D. Lundberg, "Business and Professionalism in Medicine at the American Medical Association," *Journal of the American Medical Association* 279 (1998): 169–70.

2. R. L. Cruess, S. R. Cruess, and S. E. Johnston, "Professionalism and Medicine's Social Contract," *Journal of Bone and Joint Surgery* 82 (2000): 1189–94.

3. Members of the Medical Professionalism Project, "Medical Professionalism in the New Millennium: A Physician Charter," *Annals of Internal Medicine* 136 (2002): 243–46.

4. Angell, "Is Academic Medicine for Sale?" Angell, "The Pharmaceutical Industry"; Angell, *The Truth about the Drug Companies;* Kassirer, "Academic Medical Centers under Siege"; Kassirer, *On the Take;* J. Abramson, *Overdosed America: The Broken Promise of American Medicine* (New York: HarperCollins, 2004); S. M. Wolfe, "The Destruction of Medicine by Market Forces: Teaching Acquiescence or Resistance and Change?" *Academic Medicine* 77 (2002): 5–7.

5. A. Stone, "Bright Future in Pharma Outsourcing," *Forbes July 29,* 2005, www.forbes.com/strategies/2005/07/29/covance-charles-river-pharma-cz_as_0729sf.html (Accessed April 7, 2006); A. Lustgarten, "Drug Testing Goes Offshore: Nearly 40% of All Clinical Trials Are Now Conducted in Poorer Countries Such as Russia and India, where Costs Are Lower and Patients More Vulnerable," *Fortune* August 8, 2005, 67–72. money.cnn.com/magazines/fortune/fortune_archive/2005/08/08/8267653/index.htm (Accessed April 7, 2006)

6. Red Herring, "India Emerges as New Drug Trial Hot Spot: Biotech Entrepreneurs See Indian Clinical Trials—Which Can Cut Costs by 60 percent—as the Difference between Success and Slow Death 2003," www.redherring.com/article.aspx?f = Articles/2003%2F10%2F6a1187ce-f446-434f-9b36-0379c15dac24%2F6a1187ce-f446-434f-9b36-0379c15dac24.xml&hed = India%20emerges%20as%20new%20drug%20trial%20hot%20spot (accessed August 4, 2005).

7. S. C. Gad, *The Selection and Use of Contract Research Organizations* (New York: Taylor & Francis, 2003); K. A. Getz and J. Vogel, "Achieving Results with CROs: Their Evolving Role in Clinical Development," *Applied Clinical Trials* 4 (1995): 32–38.

8. J. Yen, "Stock Focus: Pharmaceutical Research Companies," 2001, www.forbes.com/2001/06/22/0622sf.html (accessed August 4, 2005).

9. Gad, *The Selection and Use of Contract Research Organizations;* E. S. Browning, "Change in Health Care Shakes up the Business of Drug Development: Testing Now Is Often Done by 'Study Mills' Able to Underbid Universities: Contractors Supervise Trials," *Wall Street Journal,* March 28, 1995; A. Alger, "Trials and Tribulations: The Drug Revolution Could Run into a Brick Wall: Not Enough Guinea Pigs," *Forbes,* May 1999, 316–17; L. Huber, R. Drucker, and G. Hughes, *Outsourcing in Clinical Drug Development* (Boca Raton, FL: CRC Press, 2002); V. O'Connell, "Ad Agencies Join in Drug Development," *Wall Street Journal,* March 13, 2002.

10. R. Winslow, "Punishing Cure: As Both Hospital CEO and Patient, One Man Feels Drug-Price Pinch," *Wall Street Journal,* November 19, 1998.

11. R. Zimmerman, "Desperately Seeking Kids for Clinical Trials," *Wall Street Journal,* May 29, 2002.

12. Browning, "Change in Health Care."

13. Angell, "Is Academic Medicine for Sale?" J. S. Cohen, *Over Dose: The Case against the Drug Companies: Prescription Drugs, Side Effects, and Your Health* (New York: Penguin, 2001).

14. K. Eichenwald and G. Kolata, "Research for Hire: Drug Trials Hide Conflicts for Doctors," part 1, *New York Times,* May 11, 1999, www.nytimes.com/library/national/science/health/051699drug-trials.html (accessed August 4, 2005); Eichenwald and Kolata, "Research for Hire," part 2, *New York Times,* May 11, 1999, www.nytimes.com/library/national/science/health/051699drug-trials-2.html (accessed August 4, 2005); A. S. Relman and M. Angell, "America's Other Drug Problem: How the Drug Industry Distorts Medicine and Politics," *New Republic,* December 16, 2002, S27–S41.

15. C. H. Deutsch, "Scientific Solution to Save Your Skin," *New York Times,* June 13, 2003, www.nytimes.com/2003/07/13/business/yourmoney/13COSM.html?th (accessed August 4, 2005).

16. S. Beatty, "New Wrinkle: Hot at the Mall: Skin-Care Products from Physicians: 'Cosmeceutical' Creams Tap Anti-aging Market," *Wall Street Journal,* November 14, 2003.

17. J. Kaufman, "First Do No Harm: Second, Peddle a Box of All-Fabric Bleach— Doctors Upset Over Lower Pay are Selling Amway Products: Not Everyone Gets Rich," *Wall Street Journal,* June 18, 1997.

18. D. Gianelli, "Physicians as Sales Reps? Involvement in Multilevel Programs Raise Ethical Concerns," *American Medical News,* May 11, 1997, www.ama-assn.org/amed news/1997/pick_97/pick1124.htm (accessed August 4, 2005).

19. J. H. Prager, "Selling Products OK—but Not for Profit: Delegates Overrode Concerns that They Were 'Micromanaging' Medical Practice in Approving Ethical Guidelines for the Sale of Health Products from Physicians' Offices," *American Medical News,* July 12, 1999, www.ama-assn.org/amednews/1999/pick_99/prl20712.htm (accessed August 4, 2005).

20. C. Gorman, "Bleak days for doctors: The AMA Flap Isn't All That's Amiss: Physicians Are Fed up, Dropping out and Even Selling Amway," *Time,* February 8, 1999, 53.

21. S. Findlay, "Sunbeam Deal Is Downfall of Top AMA Executive," *USA Today,* December 5, 1997; S. Findlay, "AMA Rethinks Endorsing Line of Consumer Goods," *USA Today,* August 20, 1997; P. K. Harral, "If AMA Endorsement Isn't about Money, then What Is It About?" *Duluth News Tribune,* August 20, 1997.

22. Relman and Lundberg, "Business and Professionalism"; J. P. Kassirer and M. Angell, "The High Price of Product Endorsement," *New England Journal of Medicine* 337 (1997): 750; G. D. Lundberg, "The Business and Professionalism of Medicine," *Journal of the American Medical Association* 278 (1997): 1703.

23. American Medical Association. "Principles of Medical Ethics," 2001, www.ama assn.org/ama/pub/category/2512.html (accessed August 4, 2005).

24. American Medical Association. "Declaration of Professional Responsibility Medicine's Social Contract with Humanity," 2003, www.ama-assn.org/ama/pub/category/7491.html (accessed August 4, 2005).

25. R. T. King, "Bitter Pill: How a Drug Firm Paid for University Study: Then Undermined It," *Wall Street Journal,* April 12, 1996; D. Vergano, "Filed under F (for Forgotten): Drug Companies Send Unfavorable Research to the Nether Regions," *USA Today*, May 17, 2001; J. Lexchin, L. A. Bero, B. Djulbegovic, and O. Clark, "Pharmaceutical Industry Sponsorship and Research Outcome and Quality: Systematic Review," *British Medical Journal* 326 (2003): 1167–70; H. Melander, J. Ahlqvist-Rastad, G. Meijer, and B. Beermann, "Evidence B(i)ased Medicine: Selective Reporting from Studies Sponsored by Pharmaceutical Industry: Review of Studies in New Drug Applications," *British Medical Journal* 326 (2003): 1171–73.

26. American Medical Association, "Code of Medical Ethics: Current Opinions with Annotations," 2004, www.ama-assn.org/apps/pf_new/pf_online?category = CEJA&assn = AMA&f ...n = mSearch&s_t = &st_p = &nth = 1& (accessed August 4, 2005).

27. See section 8.063: "Sale of Health-Related Products from Physicians' Offices," www.ama-assn.org/apps/pf_new/pf_online?f_n = browse&doc = policyfiles/Hn E/E-8.063 .HTM&&s_t = &st_p = &nth = 1&prev_pol = policyfiles/HnE/E-7.0 5. HTM&nxt_pol − policyfiles/HnE/E-8.01.HTM& (accessed August 4, 2005).

28. Section 8.063: "Sale of Health-Related Products from Physicians' Offices."

29. American College of Physicians, "Ethics Manual: Fourth Edition," *Annals of Internal Medicine* 142 (2005): 560–82.

30. American College of Physicians, "Ethics Manual: Fourth Edition," 1999, www .annals.org/cgi/content/full/128/7/576?maxtoshow = &HITS = 10&hits = 10&RESULT FORMAT = &fulltext = %22professional + misconduct%22&searchid = 1073244177331_ 1760&stored_search = &FIRSTINDEX = 0&journalcode = annintmed (accessed August 4, 2005).

31. J. Avorn, M. Chen, and R. Hartley, "Scientific versus Commercial Sources of Influence on the Prescribing Behavior of Physicians," *American Journal of Medicine* 73 (1982): 4–8; S. Coyle, "Physician-Industry Relations. Part 1: Individual Physicians," *Annals of Internal Medicine* 136 (2002): 396–402; B. Goodman, "Do Drug Company Promotions Influence Physician Behavior?" *Western Journal of Medicine* 174 (2001): 232–33; D. Guldal and S. Semin, "The Influence of Drug Companies' Advertising Programs on Physicians," *International Journal of Health Services* 30 (2002): 585–95; M. M. Mello, M. Rosenthal, and P. J. Neumann, "Direct-to-Consumer Advertising and Shared Liability for Pharmaceutical Manufacturers," *Journal of the American Medical Association* 289 (2003): 477–81.

32. Federation of State Medical Boards. *A Guide to the Essentials of a Modern Medical Practice,* 10th ed., 2004, www.fsmb.org (accessed August 4, 2005). Section 9: "Disciplinary Action against Licensees: Grounds for Action."

33. Members of the Medical Professionalism Project, "Medical Professionalism in the New Millennium."

34. Members of the Medical Professionalism Project, "Medical Professionalism in the New Millennium."

35. For internal criticism, see P. E. Dans, J. P. Weiner, and S. E. Otter, "Peer Review Organizations: Promises and Potential Pitfalls," *New England Journal of Medicine* 313 (1985): 1131–37; F. D. Scutchfield and R. Benjamin, "The Role of the Medical Profession in Physician Discipline," *Journal of the American Medical Association* 279 (1998): 1915–16; S. M. Wolfe, "Bad Doctors Get a Free Ride," *New York Times,* March 4, 2003. For external criticism, see E. Freidson, *Profession of Medicine: A Study of the Sociology of Applied Knowledge* (New York: Harper & Row, 1970); F. W. Hafferty and D. W. J. Light, "Professional Dynamics and the Changing Nature of Medical Work," *Journal of Health and Social Behavior* 1995:132–53; F. W. Hafferty and J. B. McKinlay, *The Changing Medical Profession: An International Perspective* (New York: Oxford University Press, 1993).

36. D. A. Davis, G. R. Norman, A. Painvin, E. Lindsay, M. S. Ragbeer, and D. Rath, "Attempting to Ensure Physician Competence," *Journal of the American Medical Association* 263 (1990): 2041–42; C. Dehlendorf and S. M. Wolfe, "Physicians Disciplined for Sex-Related Offenses," *Journal of the American Medical Association* 279 (1998): 1883–88; J. Goodwin, K. Bemmann, and J. Zwieg, "Physician Sexual Exploitation: Wisconsin in the 1980s," *Journal of the American Medical Women's Association* 49 (1994): 19–23; P. Jesilow, G. Gels, and H. Pontell, "Fraud by Physicians against Medicaid," *Journal of the American Medical Association* 266 (1991): 3318–22; J. Morrison and P. Wickersham, "Physicians Disciplined by a State Medical Board," *Journal of the American Medical Association* 279 (1998): 1889–93; W. B. Schwartz and D. N. Mendelson, "Physicians Who Have Lost Their Malpractice Insurance: Their Demographic Characteristics and the Surplus-Lines Companies That Insure Them," *Journal of the American Medical Association* 262 (1989):1335–41; A. A. Skolnick, "Prison Deaths Spotlight How Boards Handle Impaired, Disciplined Physicians," *Journal of the American Medical Association* 280 (1998): 1387–90.

37. W. E. McAuliffe, M. Rohman, S. Santangelo, B. Feldman, E. Magnuson, A. Sobol, J. Weissman, "Psychotropic Drug Use among Practicing Physicians and Medical Students," *New England Journal of Medicine* 315 (1986): 805–10; P. G. O'Connor and A. Spickard Jr., "Physician Impairment by Substance Abuse (Review)," *Medical Clinic of North America* 81 (1997): 1037–52; J. H. Shore, "The Oregon Experience with Impaired Physicians on Probation: An Eight-Year Follow-Up," *Journal of the American Medical Association* 257 (1987): 2931–34.

38. Goodwin, Bemmann, and Zwieg, "Physician Sexual Exploitation"; R. B. Schmitt, "Maker of Ritalin, Psychiatric Group Sued," *Wall Street Journal,* September 14, 2001; S. H. Johnson, "Judicial Review of Disciplinary Action for Sexual Misconduct in the Practice of Medicine," *Journal of the American Medical Association* 270 (1993): 1596–1600; S. M. Wolfe, "Doctors Sanctioned for Sex Offenses Still Practicing: Hundreds of Physicians Disciplined for Sex Offenses Involving Patients," 1998, www.citizen.org/pressroom/release.cfm?ID = 934 (accessed August 4, 2005).

39. For California, see Morrison and Wickersham, "Physicians Disciplined." For Ohio, see S. W. Clay and R. R. Conatser, "Characteristics of Physicians Disciplined by the State

Medical Board of Ohio," *Journal of the American Osteopathic Association* 103 (2003): 81–88.

40. R. Pear, "Inept Physicians Are Rarely Listed as Law Requires," *New York Times,* May 29, 2001, http://query.nytimes.com/gst/fullpage.html?sec = health&res = 9906E7D 7153CF93A A15756C0A9679C8B63 (accessed April 7, 2006); "HMOs Give Bad Doctors a Pass, Put Patients at Risk: 84% Reported May 28, 2001, Nothing to National Databank in Past Decade," *USA Today,* May 31, 2001; Wolfe, "Bad Doctors Get a Free Ride"; C. J. Gearon, "Unmasking Unsafe Doctors: The Info Is There, but You Have to Dig," 2001, www.aarp.org/bulletin/yourhealth/Articles/a2003-08-07-unmasking.html (accessed August 4, 2005).

41. L. Landro, "Has Your Doctor Been Sued? New Laws Allow Patients to Check Criminal Records, Disciplinary Actions Online," *Wall Street Journal,* July 18, 2002

42. Public Citizen, www.citizen.org, 2005 (accessed August 4, 2005).

43. S. D. Smith, "Group Pans MN Doc Discipline: Nader Group Says Too Little Punishment," *Business Journal,* April 22, 2002, www.bizjournals.com/twincities/stories/2002/04/22/story5.html (accessed August 10, 2005); S. Lundine, "Medical Board Still Falls Short in Doc Discipline," *Business Journal,* April 17, 2000, orlando.bizjournals.com/orlando/stories/2000/04/17/story2.html (accessed August 4, 2005); S. Lundine, "Low Ratings a Bitter Pill for Medical Board," *Business Journal,* May 14, 2001, www.biz journals.com/southflorida/stories/2001/05/14/story7.html?jst = s_cnehl (accessed August 4, 2005); "Missouri, Kansas Rank Well for Disciplinary Actions against Doctors," *Business Journal,* March 11, 2003, www.bizjournals.com/kansascity/stories/2003/11/03/daily 46.html?jst = s_rs_ hl (accessed August 4, 2005).

44. For a common Web site from which to access all state boards, as well as the individual state rankings by Public Citizen, see www.citizen.org/hrg/forms/medicalboard.cfm (accessed August 4, 2005).

45. Links to all state medical boards can be found on the AMA site at "Links to State Medical Boards." See www.ama-assn.org/ama/pub/category/2645.html (accessed August 4, 2005).

46. Alaska state board, www.dced.state.ak.us/occ/pmed.htm (accessed August 4, 2005).

47. Arizona state board, www.bomex.org (accessed August 4, 2005).

48. Arkansas state board, www.armedicalboard.org/index.asp (accessed August 4, 2005).

49. Arkansas state board, www.armedicalboard.org/index.asp (accessed August 4, 2005).

50. California state board, www.medbd.ca.gov (accessed August 4, 2005).

51. Federation of State Medical Boards, www.fsmb.org (accessed August 4, 2005).

52. Public Citizen's national database can be accessed at www.questionabledoctors.org (accessed August 4, 2005).

53. L. Arnold, "Assessing Professional Behavior: Yesterday, Today, and Tomorrow," *Academic Medicine* 77 (2002): 502–15; D. Stern, *Measuring Professionalism* (New York: Oxford University Press, 2005).

5

After *Cheng* (Sincerity): The Professional Ethics of Traditional Chinese Medicine

Jing-Bao Nie

A listing of a few of the distinctive concepts, theories, procedures, techniques, and treatments developed by traditional Chinese Medicine (TCM) over many centuries suggests the apparent differences between this medical system and modern biomedicine originating in the West: *yin-yang*, the five phases or agents, *qi*, essence, the five viscera and six bowels, channels and points, tongue-observing, moxibustion, "damp heat affecting the spleen," "exhausted fire of the middle burners," "extinguishing wind by nourishing yin," "treating cold with cold and treating heat with heat," "white tiger decoction," and "cockcrow powder." To modern sensibilities—with the exception of a handful of individuals who have consistently romanticized ancient or foreign ideas and practices—these terms sound primitive, unscientific, exotic, strange, or even laughable. Even many contemporary Chinese do not feel at home with these "old-fashioned" concepts. Nevertheless, TCM undeniably works in practice for at least some illness or diseases (e.g., the use of acupuncture to relieve certain kinds of chronic pain), despite the inability of modern science to explain adequately the nature of the "channels" and "points" involved. It works—regardless of the foreign character of its concepts and theories for patients—just as contemporary biomedicine works even though those who are sick have no real knowledge of anatomy, physiology, or pathology. Other ancient medical traditions, like those of Greece and Rome, are today merely part of history, supplanted by more effective treatments. Yet TCM is still alive today as one of the main healing systems practiced extensively in East Asia side by side with modern biomedicine. Even in the West, the techniques of TCM—a cornerstone of the developing field of complementary and alternative medicine—are increasingly by patients accepted as a fresh alternative approach.

As TCM evolved in China, its practitioners formulated a series of pragmatic rules governing the physician's decorum. Moreover, in an effort to systematize their occupational morality according to the key concepts of Chinese ethical-social worldviews, they put forward some core principles of professional ethics, including the concepts of the virtuous physician (*liangyi*), medicine as the art of humanity or humaneness (*yi nai renshu*), sincerity or moral excellence (*cheng*), and compassion (*ci*). Although the Chinese concepts of professional ethics may not seem as strange as some of the corresponding medical terms, it is far from clear that they will be able to continue to serve as guides for practice today. In this age of globalization and Western hegemony, it is far from certain whether the professional ethics of TCM can serve as a source of inspiration for promoting a more ethically rooted practice of medicine and a deeper concept of professionalism—or even if it can survive as the moral foundation for practitioners of TCM in China and elsewhere. At a time when TCM continues to be a major medical system in the East and is serving more people in the West, the vitality of traditional Chinese medical ethics is being threatened, if not completely lost.

There are complex sociocultural and intellectual obstacles that prevent us from taking seriously the professional ethics of TCM and recognizing its contemporary significance. Three factors stand out. First is the Western habit of treating Chinese traditions as strange, unscientific, and parochial. Second is the trend in both contemporary Chinese and Western scholarship that equates traditional Chinese medical ethics merely with decorum, a set of good behaviors displayed by the individual physician and nothing more. A third factor, and one with particular significance in the Chinese context, is a nihilistic modernist perspective that categorizes the past as backward, primitive, an obstacle to progress, and something that should be discarded. In the twentieth century, China developed a wholesale antitraditionalism that first became prominent in the May Fourth movement and reached its peak in the notorious Cultural Revolution. Just as Chinese traditions like Confucianism were viewed as an obstacle to modernization and, at best, irrelevant to modern China's search for national strength, wealth, and power, traditional Chinese medical ethics is regarded as having only a very limited or supplementary role in contemporary health-care practice.

This chapter aims to offer an introduction to the professional ethics of TCM through a study of the most influential document of Chinese medical ethics, the *Lun Dayi Jingcheng* (On the Proficiency and Sincerity of the Master Physician) of the great seventh-century physician Sun Simaio (Sun Szu-miao). To better explain the professional ethics of TCM as articulated by Sun, I will also sketch out some of the metaphysical and spiritual dimensions of Chinese medical professionalism by presenting the multiple layers of Confucian understandings of *cheng*, often but inadequately translated as "sincerity," but also meaning authenticity, purity, honesty, genuineness, truth, reality, self-realization, and moral excellence. While contemporary Chinese and Western scholars[1] have treated humanity or humaneness (*ren*, often perceived as the core notion of Confucian ethics and politics) and/or compassion (*ci*, a key ethical concept from Buddhism) as *the* basic principle of traditional Chinese medical ethics, this chapter focuses on the notion of *cheng* (sincerity), which in my view constitutes the core doctrine of professionalism of TCM, especially when it is concerned about the personal morality of practitioners.

THE MEDICAL PROFESSION AND PROFESSIONAL ETHICS IN CHINA

For sociologists, the concept of profession implies far more than an ordinary occupation. According to Eliot Freidson, an occupation becomes a formal profession only when it obtains legitimate and organized autonomy, that is, the right to control its own work in an exclusive way and freedom from supervision by society.[2] Medicine in the United States since the Flexner Report, and especially since World War II, constitutes the archetype of professionalism in this sociological perspective. Under the criteria for professions developed in the United States, the process of professionalization of medicine in China did not truly begin until the twentieth century, when modern Western biomedicine took root in China and began to marginalize TCM and other traditional healing systems. Under the threefold spell of scientism, modernism, and radical anti-traditionalism, proposals were made and actions taken to abolish TCM in the first half of the twentieth century in China.[3] In the case of TCM, the beginnings of professionalization can be viewed as a response to a threat to its survival. In fact, as a result of its specific sociopolitical contexts, even in contemporary China medicine—whether TCM or biomedicine—hardly enjoys the kind of autonomy that characterizes the American medical profession.

Despite the recent professionalization of TCM, some elements necessary for the development of a profession are detectable in early Chinese civilization. First among these elements is the systematized body of knowledge of TCM, with foundations reaching back to the Han dynasty (205 B.C.E. to 220

C.E.) or even earlier. These foundations include the appearance in this period of the so-called "four classics" of TCM, comprising the two theoretical volumes *Huangdi Neijing* (The Yellow Emperor's Classic of Medicine, which consists of two parts, *Suwen* and *Lingxu*) and *Nan Jing* (The Classic of Difficult Issues), as well as clinical works such as *Shanghan Zabing Lun* (On Various Fevers and Internal Diseases) and *Shennong Bencao Jing* (The Legendary Farmer's Classic of Materia Medica). According to the *Huangdi Neijing*, in remote and supposedly "golden" antiquity, physicians were obliged to participate in a set of rituals and take an oath sworn in blood before beginning the study and practice of acupuncture.[4] Unfortunately, no surviving historical works have recorded how the rituals were performed nor the content of the oath. The second element of a growing profession observed in Chinese history is the division of labor and specialization which occurred as early as the third century B.C.E., when the imperial palace had specialists in medical administration, nutrition, internal medicine, and surgery.[5] Third, the governance and regulation of practitioners within a national system of medical education and qualifying examinations began, at least for physicians in the imperial court, over fifteen hundred years ago. State-sponsored medical services and state-controlled medical education evolved together early in the history of China.[6] The fourth and most telling aspect of the development of professionalism was the creation of a distinctive professional ethics in TCM.

Normally, each medical system has its own professional morality or ethics. Rooted in the sociocultural and historical context in which a given medical system originated and grew, the resulting professional ethics can vary from rules of thumb based on the practitioners' customs to a systematic professionalism. Although professional medical ethics usually develop alongside the process of professionalizing the services of healers, a formal profession is not required for the existence of a professional ethics. And while professional ethics may not be the crucial and necessary attribute of a formal profession, as medical sociologists have argued, they are essential for the mature development of any profession.

Since antiquity, many discussions on moral issues in medicine, including consideration of the professional behavior of practitioners, have appeared in a variety of works, such as those by physicians like Zhang Zhongjing, philosophers like Confucius and Lie Zi, and historians like Sima Qian. One of the most notable essays was *Lun Yi* (On the Physician) from the *Wuli Lun* (A Treatise on the Nature of Things) by Yang Quan, a fourth-century scholar. For Yang, the practice of medicine requires not only talent, intelligence, knowledge, and the requisite skills, but above all virtue and moral character. One should not seek medical help from those lacking in humanity and universal love (*boai*) and should not entrust oneself to practitioners without wisdom and a well-cultivated morality. He distinguishes the "good" or excellent physician (*liangyi*) from the "celebrated" one (*mingyi*) and points out that the latter does not necessarily imply the former, for even a nameless doctor can be excellent. He gives high praise to the ancient tradition in which only those who displayed both natural talent and excellent moral character were selected by the community to study and practice the art of medicine.[7]

This insistence on a high standard of both expertise and morality is again the central theme of the seventh-century paradigmatic writings of Sun Simaio on professional ethics. In fact, the emphasis on excellence in both the professional skills and moral character of the physician constitutes the basis of the professional ethics of TCM. After Sun, many writers expanded discussions on medical behavior and ethical practice, including material likely to be relevant to practitioners in the twenty-first century. I list a few well-known authors and texts here. Zhang Gao (c. 1149–1227), a Confucian physician heavily influenced by Buddhism, expressed his views on the ethics of medical practice and the development of morally good physicians in his *Yishuo* (Teachings on Medicine). Zhang offered his teachings in a series of anecdotes and stories intended to promote right action, such as not performing abortions. In the sixteenth century, the physician Zhu Huiming introduced particular topics such as "Physicians Should Preserve Humaneness," "Good Conduct Brings Reward," and "The Importance of Determining the Prospects for a Good or Bad Cure at an Early Stage." Gong Tingxian, a prolific medical writer of the seventeenth century employed by the Imperial Office for Medicine, offered his "Ten Maxims for Physicians" and, in a suggestion of mutual ethical obligations, "Ten Maxims for Patients." In the same century, Chen Shigong authored the classic *Waike Zhengzong* (Orthodox Manual of Surgery) with chapters including "Five Admonitions to Physicians" and "Ten Maxims for Physicians."[8]

A couple of caveats. First, although the works of the classical medical authors of China might suggest a unified system, the diversity of medical practice in China cannot be overemphasized. It is important to notice that there is no single Chinese culture, morality, healing system, definitive Chinese medical ethics, archetypical Chinese medical practitioner, or singular moral discourse for a wide range of practitioners.[9] Second, it is unclear what influence these maxims and admonitions had on daily medical practice or the character of medical practitioners. Historically speaking, as many medical ethics authors repeatedly complained and deplored, many physicians were not that ethical, and only a few truly good or enlightened.

PURSUING PROFICIENCY AND SINCERITY: THE
IDEAL OF TECHNICAL AND MORAL EXCELLENCE

The *Lun Dayi Jingcheng* (On the Proficiency and Sincerity of the Master Physician),[10] a chapter of the monumental medical work *Beiji Qianjin Yaofang* (Prescriptions Worth More Than a Thousand Pieces of Gold) (often abbreviated as Qianjin Yaofang), was written by Sun Simiao (c. 581–682) in the early Tang dynasty. It is considered the most important document of medical ethics in Chinese history and has had enormous influence, with a status similar to that of the Hippocratic Oath in the West. Sun brought together medical practice and techniques known prior to the seventh century, and his work served as a guide for practitioners in later centuries in China, Japan, Korea, and elsewhere in East Asia. He is known as "the king of medicine" among the populace. His life and achievements have made him a paradigm of ethical practice and elevated him to the position of the ideal physician, not only because of the high standard of morality advocated in his medical ethics writing, but also because he was known to have met these standards in his own medical practice. Even his longevity (Sun lived to 101) is treated as a symbol of his great virtue and humaneness because Confucianism considers longevity a fruit of virtuous life.

The key tenet of Sun's ethics, as the title of this important text indicates, is that a physician must be simultaneously *jing* (proficient, or at least competent, in the study and practice of medicine) and *cheng* (sincere in one's moral commitment, honest, and virtuous). Sun Simaio was the first to put forward the ideal of *dayi* (the Master Physician) and to articulate the ethical principles and manners appropriate to the role. Beginning with insightful discussions on how to learn and master the art of medicine, the *Lun Dayi Jingcheng* focuses on the professional ethics of medical practice.[11]

Like other classic medical authors such as those of *Huangdi Neijing*, Sun starts by emphasizing the difficulty of learning medicine, first by citing an earlier scholar. The study of medicine requires devotion and tenacity. It is dangerous "to pursue the most subtle matters with the most careless and superficial studies." "Only those who learn with the heart and study meticulously" can begin to understand the complexity and subtlety of medicine. Sun strongly opposes the habit of being satisfied with a smattering of knowledge on a particular subject (*qianchang jizhi*, stopping after gaining a little knowledge of something). Any true student of medicine must "master all the sources of medicine and study them diligently and constantly" (*boji yiyuan, jingqing buzhuan*). Even those who study in this way may not achieve excellence in medicine because there is the need for more than human insight. For Sun, medicine, like divination, involves grasping the finest subtleties with the help of "divine revelation," something beyond purely human talent and power.

In the *Lun Dayi Xiye* (On the Master Physician's Way of Learning Medicine), another chapter in his masterwork *Qianjin Yaofang*, Sun discusses in detail the proper course of study entailed in becoming a physician. To be competent in the art of medicine, one must first have a substantial general education. A thorough knowledge of the ancient classics and of history, literature, and philosophy is essential. Thus Confucianism, Daoism, and other schools of thought, as well as astrology and divination, are appropriate premedical subjects. One must also study the classic works of medicine, acupuncture, and materia medica. Finally, learning must not only come from books. One must practice the arts one studies and acquire personal experience as a physician, because the knowledge derived from books is never sufficient.

Jing refers to excellence not only in medical skills but also in personal morality. In the *Lun Dayi Jingcheng*, Sun formulates the fundamental ethical principles of healing and elaborates the moral excellence of the Master Physician. A good physician must first of all cultivate a heart of genuine and deep compassion for human pain, suffering, and distress:

> When a Master Physician practices medicine, he must calm his mind . . . develop a heart of great mercy and compassion, and solemnly pledge to relieve without any discrimination the pains from which the souls of all existences (*hunling*)—human beings suffer.

Sun promotes a universal medical humanism and maintains that a doctor should treat all patients equally:

> When the ill come for help, whether they are noble or lowly, rich or poor, old or young, handsome or homely, enemies or good friends, Chinese or foreigners, intelligent or simple minded, the Master Physician should pay no attention to any of these things but rather should treat all his patients equally, as if they were his closest relatives.

For Sun, a morally excellent physician takes a heroic attitude toward medicine. He stresses that a physician should not shrink back from his work because of an unfavorable or even dangerous situation but should instead always involve himself wholeheartedly.

> A physician should not be overcautious and indecisive, should not worry about good or bad luck, and should not be concerned about his own body and life. Seeing the patient unwell, a physician should feel as if he himself had been struck down. With deep sympathy welling up from the bottom of his heart, a physician should not merely appear to have done his best but get involved wholeheartedly—not worrying

whether the location is dangerous and precipitous, the time is day or night, the weather cold or hot, or whether he himself is hungry, thirsty and exhausted. Whoever practices medicine in this way is a Master Physician to all human beings. Whoever practices medicine in a contrary way is the worst enemy of humankind.

As a result, a good doctor should never shrink from treating a patient who suffers from a loathsome illness like skin ulcers:

Among the patients will be those suffering from skin ulcers and foul-smelling dysentery whom no one wants to examine, and others hate to visit. A physician should not show even a small amount of unwillingness but treat the sick with compassion, sympathy, and pity. This is my commitment.

Most notably, Sun's view of professional ethics required a physician to treat all forms of life—animals and human alike—equally. This is a very radical viewpoint in Chinese medicine and clearly came from Sun's Buddhist beliefs. In the materia medica of TCM, a large number of drugs are derived from animal body parts. Standing alone among his peers, Sun strongly opposes this practice:

Although animals are usually devalued and humans valued, animals and humans are the same in loving their own lives. To damage others for the benefit of oneself goes against the nature of even physical things—let alone the feelings of us human beings.

Sun's principle here is that "to kill one life to save another life takes us further away from life." This is the reason that living creatures are never used to make drugs in the prescriptions in his medical book.

Sun then outlines how a virtuous doctor should behave as an individual, and especially how he should treat his patients:

The manner of a Master Physician should be concentrated on his inner self, appearing composed to others, carrying himself with ease and confidence, and behaving in neither an overbearing nor servile manner. When examining the patient and diagnosing the disease, he should pay the closest attention. He should scrutinize all the symptoms in great detail and should not err by a hair's breadth. In prescribing acupuncture or herbs, he should not be in any kind of doubt. Even though the disease should be treated as soon as possible, the physician should not be rushed in dealing with a case but should investigate it carefully and reflect on it deeply. If, to show off and gain a reputation for making a speedy diagnosis, a physician acts carelessly over matters of life and death, this is contrary to the way of humanity (*buren*).

As the major location for treatment before the advent of modern clinics and hospitals was the patient's home, Sun emphasizes that a physician should behave with decorum when attending his patients in their own homes:

After arriving at the patient's home, the physician should not look around even though his eyes are dazzled with silks and satins. He is not distracted at all, although his ears are filled with beautiful music from string and bamboo instruments. When delicious food is presented to him, one course after another, he eats as if the food had no taste. When various fine wines are offered him, he treats them as if they did not exist. The physician is to behave in this way because, when one of its members is distressed due to illness, the whole family will be unhappy—not to mention the fact that pain and suffering never leave the patient even for a moment. For the physician to simply enjoy everything and take a professional pride in himself in the patient's home shames both humans and deities, and is something the Perfect Man should never do. All this points to the true meaning of medicine.

In addition, Sun strongly advises that a good physician should not talk too much, never boast about his own achievements and virtues, and never belittle his colleagues:

Regarding the way of practicing medicine, the physician should not be talkative, nor tease people, raise his voice, gossip, judge others, parade his fame, belittle his fellow physicians, nor be conceited over his own virtue. Whenever he has treated a case successfully—perhaps by chance rather than skill—he should not put his nose in the air, puff himself up, and claim that no physician under heaven could measure up to him. That kind of behavior is the terminal illness of medical practitioners.

Citing Lao Zi (Lao Tzu), the founder of Daoism, Sun holds that visible virtuous conduct will be rewarded by humans, and invisible good deeds by the spirits, while immoral behavior—even that hidden from human eyes—will be punished supernaturally. If the medical practitioner refrains from using his skills for gaining material goods but is rather determined to relieve suffering, "he will be happy on the way to the underworld."

For Sun, a doctor should not take advantage of the vulnerability of any patient, rich or poor, in any situation:

To take another example—noticing that the patient is rich and enjoys noble status, in order to show off his rare abilities the physician then prescribes precious and expensive drugs and intentionally makes it hard for the patient to get the medicine. This is not the way of conscientiousness and altruism (*zhongxu*).

In summary, Sun Simiao stipulates moral requirements for the practice of medicine as well as making practical suggestions for the conduct of physicians. He ends his powerful and eloquent work with an apology:

As my aim is to cure and relieve sickness, I have not refrained from discussing these apparently trivial matters. Whoever studies medicine should not treat them as something vulgar and be ashamed of talking about them.

In a second major medical work, the *Qianjin Yifan* (Supplement to Prescriptions Worth a Thousand Pieces of Gold), published when he was about one hundred years old, Sun further prescribes ten types of good conduct in medical practice: 1) Assist those in need and those with difficulties; 2) Respect demons and celestial beings; 3) Do not kill or injure anyone; 4) Develop an attitude of compassion; 5) Do not envy the rich or despise the poor; 6) Cultivate a temperate disposition; 7) Avoid valuing luxurious items and despising ordinary ones; 8) Seek moderation in diet by avoiding wine, meat, and rich food; 9) Seek moderation in life and avoid indulging in women or music; and 10) Maintain a well-balanced disposition and character.[12]

In general, Sun emphasizes that the purpose of medical practice is to help others rather than gain material goods and fame. In the Confucian and Buddhist moral and spiritual sense, he would have considered healing as a vocation or calling. At the heart of his maxims and instructions on learning and practicing medicine, *cheng* (sincerity of moral commitment or moral excellence in general) is the foundation and first principle of Sun's professionalism. *Cheng* is the starting point of medical practice, for only those who are sincere in their moral commitment will study medicine diligently and tirelessly, move divines and thus master the art. Here, the notion of *cheng*, as demonstrated in the Confucian tradition, is not only psychological, implying a unity between actions and beliefs, but metaphysical, religious, and spiritual as well.

CHENG IN CONFUCIANISM: THE PHILOSOPHICAL AND SPIRITUAL BASIS OF TRADITIONAL CHINESE PROFESSIONAL ETHICS

While traditional Chinese medical ethics has been influenced most heavily by Confucianism, there are also significant elements derived from Buddhism and Daoism. Indeed, Sun Simaio's *Lun Dayi Jingcheng* is an eclectic product of elements drawn from Confucianism, Buddhism, and Daoism. All three of these major social and ethical traditions of imperial China emphasize the importance of sincerity in moral life. The classic Confucian discussion of *cheng* comes from the *Zhongyong*, often translated as *The Doctrine of the Mean*, which is one of the canonical "Four Books" in Confucianism. According to historians of Chinese philosophy, the teachings of the *Zhongyan* attracted both Buddhists and Daoists even before neo-Confucianism put it as one of a few most fundamental Confucian works.[13] Scholars from these differing, and sometimes conflicting, traditions wrote their own commentaries on the *Zhongyong* from rather early times. The idea of sincerity as the heart of the moral life is appealing to both Buddhist and Daoist traditions, despite their differences from Confucian thought in other areas.

In the eleventh century, the neo-Confucian philosopher Zhou Dengyi (Chou Tun-i) placed *cheng* (sincerity) as the foundation of all the virtues:

> Sagehood is nothing but sincerity. It is the foundation of the Five Constant Virtues (humanity, righteousness, propriety, wisdom, and faithfulness) and the source of all activities. . . . Without sincerity, the Five Constant Virtues and all activities will be wrong. They will be depraved and obstructed. Therefore with sincerity very little effort is needed [to achieve the Mean]. [In itself] it is perfectly easy but it is difficult to put into practice. But with determination and firmness, there will be no difficulty. . . . It is [a] subtle, incipient, activating force giving rise to good and evil.[14]

For Sun Simiao, sincerity is the foundation of other virtues needed for learning and practicing medicine, including persistence, medical humanism, medical heroism, treating all patients equally, and respecting all forms of life.

Psychologically, sincerity entails both avoiding cheating others and not indulging in self-deception. It means behaving honestly with others and being honest with oneself. The *Daxue* (The Great Learning), the first of the "Four Books" of Confucianism, defines "making the will sincere" as one of the eight steps toward the acquisition of wisdom and becoming a sage:

> What is meant by "making the will sincere" is allowing no self-deception, as when we hate a bad smell or love a beautiful color. . . . For other people see him [a sincere individual] as if they see his very heart. This is what is meant by saying that what is true in a man's heart will be shown in his outward appearance. Therefore the superior man will always be watchful with himself when alone. . . . Wealth makes a house shine and virtue makes a person shine. When one's mind is broad and one's heart generous, one's body becomes big and is at ease. Therefore the superior man will always make his will sincere.[15]

For Sun Simiao, those who believe that they have already achieved technical and moral excellence in medicine are deceiving themselves about the nature of the art and oneself.

The notion that sincerity is about how one behaves even when unobserved, and about a unity of knowing and acting, suggests a psychological aspect to this concept. But sincerity is not just a state of mind, for it also implies a state of being and thus has a metaphysical and religious character. The *Zhongyong* itself links sincerity with not only growth in virtue and human responsibility, but spirituality ("heaven") and Dao (the Way) as well:

> Sincerity is the Way of heaven. To think how to be sincere is the way of man. He who is sincere is one who hits upon what is right without effort and apprehends

without thinking. He is naturally and easily in harmony with the Way. Such a man is a sage. He who tries to be sincere is one who chooses the good and holds fast to it. . . . Study it [the way to be sincere] extensively, inquire into it accurately, think over it carefully, sift it clearly, and practice earnestly. When there is anything not yet studied, or studied but not yet understood, do not give up. . . . If another man succeeds by one effort, you will use a hundred efforts. If another man succeeds by ten efforts, you will use a thousand efforts. If one really follows this course, though stupid, he will surely become intelligent, and, though weak, will surely become strong.[16]

The key insight of the Confucian moral understanding and vision of *cheng* is that only those who are absolutely sincere can fully develop their nature. The infinite purity of sincerity cannot but reveal itself. Interestingly, according to Chan, a modern compiler and commentator on Chinese philosophical texts, the five steps involved in following the way of sincerity—study, inquiry, thinking, sifting, and practice—resemble the educational philosophy of John Dewey.[17]

Moreover, *cheng* is not only a state of being but also a process of becoming and self-completion. As Tu Wei-ming, a brilliant contemporary Confucian scholar, points out, "*Ch'eng* as a state of being signifies the ultimate reality of human nature and, as a process of becoming, the necessary way of actualizing that reality in concrete, ordinary human affairs. Therefore, *ch'eng* symbolizes not only what a person in an ultimate sense ought to be but also what a person in a concrete way can eventually become."[18] In the case of medicine, the Master Physician embodies this state of being and this process of becoming.

In his groundbreaking study of medical ethics in imperial China, Paul Unschuld explores the role of ethics in the way practitioners develop their profession. Unschuld defines professionalization as "the process by which one group (or a number of them) endeavors to expand its possession of the medically related resources available in a culture, until it exercises exclusive control over those resources." From Unschuld's sociological perspective the development of professional ethics, even those based on sincerity and authenticity, is still a manifestation of self-interest. Unschuld's insightful thesis on the origin of professional ethics in China echoes the remark of the fourth-century B.C.E. philosopher and social thinker Hanfei Zi: "Physicians are good at sucking human sores and drawing in the diseased blood with their mouth. They do so not because they see their patients as their close family members but because this is where their profits lie and self-interests can be achieved."[19] It also echoes the well-known remark of Adam Smith on the human pursuit of self-interest: "It is not from the benevolence of the butcher, the brewer, or the baker that we expect our dinner, but from their regard to their own interest. We address ourselves, not to their humanity but to their self-love."[20] It can even remind us of the extreme cynicism of the ancient Greek comic writer who, according to Montaigne's essay "One man's profit is another man's harm," claimed that "no doctor takes pleasure in the health even of his friends."[21]

Yet Montaigne's point is to reveal the absurdity of the suggestion that making profit out of another's misfortune is morally wrong, because no profit can be made except at the expense of others. Pursuing self-interest does not contradict a sincere and authentic concern for the welfare of others. Adam Smith also acknowledges that self-interest exists alongside the beneficent aspects of human nature. In *The Theory of Moral Sentiments*, Smith states that the sentiment of "pity or compassion" exists "evidently" in all humanity, not only in the "virtuous and humane" but even in "the great ruffian," albeit in different degrees.[22]

Confucianism anticipated a similar perspective centuries earlier than Smith, although even among Confucians the question of whether human nature is intrinsically good or evil has been controversial. Mencius, one of the central sages of Confucianism, notes: "Man's nature is naturally good just as water naturally flows downward. There is no man without this good nature."[23] Humanity comes from within the heart of each individual. The Confucian roots of traditional Chinese professional ethics provide a broad platform for the notion of building on the natural goodness of human nature.

CONCLUSION

In the West, there is a recognition that the Hippocratic oath already exists to provide a source of inspiration for medical professionalism today.[24] Traditional Chinese morality likewise has a contemporary relevance and, potentially, a deeper significance (given some of the problems that afflict the medical profession) in its emphasis on sincerity, personal growth, and enlightened care of the other. A medical ethic and ethics of professionalism based on sincerity create a vision of a profession that allows for transparency of relationships, a dedication to the other as a recognition of enlightened self-interest, and a mode of being that would transform medical practice from a technical craft into a spiritual pathway.

In striking contrast with this Chinese notion of *"cheng"* is almost exclusive stress on external standards in contemporary Eastern and Western medical professionalism, the distinguishing feature and guiding spirit of which is an "ethics of rules," rather than a more traditional "ethics of character or virtue." Contemporary ethical codes of medicine—such as the series of international declarations on medical ethics, especially research ethics, by the

World Association of Medical Associations, the *Code of Medical Ethics* issued by the American Medical Association, and the "Regulation of Medical Morality for Medical Professionals in the People's Republic of China" promulgated by the Chinese Ministry of Health—are all dominated by an ethics of rules. In both the East and the West today, the issue of a practitioner's sincerity or authenticity in his or her moral commitment—whether one is "a virtuous person"—is seemingly not as important as following the rules listed in the professional codes. Rather, "acting in conformity with the rules" and "playing the role of a medical professional" are presented as far more important than the practitioner's individual moral formation. Doubtless, the rules are essential for the development of any ethically sound medical practice. And a medical ethics based on Confucianism can be compatible with the standard contemporary bioethical principles, although the way of prioritizing these principles may be significantly different.[25] Even for the professionalism of Sun Simiao the rules are extremely important. Nevertheless, in the perspective of the professional ethics of TCM based on *cheng,* contemporary theories and practice of medical professionalism have very much ignored the central role of not only the inner characteristics of the moral agent but also the metaphysical and spiritual dimension of any moral life.

NOTES

I am grateful to Dr. Kayhan Parsi for his many generous helps and Dr. Paul Sorrell for his professional assistance with the English language.

1. Ren-Zhong Qiu, "Medicine—the Art of Humaneness: On Ethics of Traditional Chinese Medicine," *Journal of Medicine and Philosophy* 13 (1): 35–73; Daqing Zhang and Zhifan Cheng, "Medicine Is a Humane Art: The Basic Principles of Professional Ethics in Chinese Medicine," *Hastings Center Report* 30 (4)(2000): S8–S12; Shui-Chuen Lee, *Rujia Shengming Lunlixue* [Confucian Bioethics] (Taipei: Ehu Press, 1999); Paul Unschuld, *Medical Ethics in Imperial China: A Study of Historical Anthropology* (Berkeley and Los Angeles: University of California Press, 1979); Albert Jonsen, *A Short History of Medical Ethics* (New York: Oxford University Press, 2000), 36–41.

2. Eliot Freidson, *Profession of Medicine* (Chicago: University of Chicago Press, 1988).

3. See Ralph C. Croizier, *Traditional Medicine in Modern China* (Cambridge, MA: Harvard University Press, 1968); Hongjun Zhao, *Jindai Zhongxiyi Lunzheng Shi* [The Modern History of the Controversies between Chinese and Westen Medicine] (Hefei: Anfei Science and Technology Press, 1989).

4. See chapters 9 and 48, Nanjing College of Chinese Medicine, *Huandi Neijing Lingshu Yishi* [Lingshu of The Yellow Emperor's Classic of Medicine: Text, Translation, and Annotations] (Shanghai: Shanghai Science and Technology Press, 1986).

5. Menglei Chen, *Gujin Tushu Jicheng Yibu Quanlu* [Collection of Ancient and Con-

temporary Books, Section on Medicine], book 12: *General Discussions,* original vols. 501–20, (Beijing: People's Health Press, 1962 [1723]), 2–3.

6. Joseph Needham, *Science and Civilization in China,* vol. 6, part 6: *Medicine,* with the collaboration of Lu Gwei-Djen and Nathan Sivin (Cambridge: Cambridge University Press, 2000).

7. Chen, *Gujin Tushu Jicheng Yibu Quanlu*: Book 12, 15.

8. For some important primary materials, see Chen, *Gujin Tushu Jicheng Yibu Quanlu*: Book 12. For secondary Chinese works, see Yimou Zhou, *Lidai Mingyi Lun Yide* (Ancient Well-known Chinese Physicians on Medical Morality) (Changsha: Hunan Science and Technology Press, 1983); Zhaoxong He, ed., *Zhongguo Yide Shi* [A History of Medical Morality in China] (Shanghai: Shanghai Medical University Press, 1988). For an English study with translation of primary materials, see Unschuld, *Medical Ethics.*

9. Jing-Bao Nie, "The Plurality of Chinese and American Medical Moralities: Toward an Interpretive Cross-Cultural Bioethics," *Kennedy Institute of Ethics Journal* (10) 3 (2000): 239–60; Jing-Bao Nie, *Behind the Silence: Chinese Voices on Abortion* (Lanham, MD: Rowman & Littlefield, 2005); Jing-Bao Nie, "The Moral Discourses of Practitioners in China," in *A History of Medical Ethics,* eds. Robert Baker and Larry McCullough (New York: Cambridge University Press, 2006).

10. Paul Unschuld translates *"dayi jingcheng"* as "the absolute sincerity of great physicians" (*Medical Ethics,* 29). In modern and classic Chinese, *"jing cheng"* usually means "absolute sincerity or total honesty," as in the set phrase *"jingcheng suo zhi, jingshi wei kai"* (total sincerity can affect even metal and stone). But here *jing* can be read also as a noun parallel to *cheng,* rather than as an adjective qualifying *cheng.* The term *jingcheng* first appeared in "The Old Fisherman," chapter 32 of *Zhuang Zi (Chuang Tzu),* the ancient Daoist classic. The text, translated by Burton Watson, reads: "By the 'Truth' I mean purity and sincerity in their highest degree. He who lacks purity and sincerity cannot move others." See Burton Watson, *The Complete Worlds of Chuang Tzu* (New York: Columbia University Press, 1968), 349.

11. Simiao Sun, *Beiji Qianjin Yaofang* (Prescriptions Worth More Than a Thousand Pieces of Gold) (Beijing: People's Health Press, 1998). The Chinese version can be easily found in many texts, including Chen, *Gujin Tushu Jicheng Yibu Quanlu,* 16–17, and Zhou 1983, 98–103. For a complete English translation, see Unschuld, *Medical Ethics,* 29–33. The translations of the text included in this chapter are mine.

12. Cited in Unschuld, *Medical Ethics,* 33–34.

13. Wing-Tsit Chan, *A Source Book in Chinese Philosophy* (Princeton, NJ: Princeton University Press, 1963), 95.

14. Chan, *A Source Book in Chinese,* 466.

15. Chan, *A Source Book in Chinese,* 90.

16. Chan, *A Source Book in Chinese,* 107.

17. Chan, *A Source Book in Chinese,* 107.

18. Wei-Ming Tu, *Centrality and Commonality: An Essay on Confucian Religiousness* (Albany: State University of New York Press, 1989), 80.

19. Chen, *Gujin Tushu Jicheng Yibu Quanlu*: Book 12, 454.

20. Adam Smith, *Wealth of Nations* (New York: Prometheus Books, 1991), 20.

21. Donald M. Frame, trans., *The Complete Essays of Montaigne* (Stanford, CA: Stanford University Press, 1965 [1958]), 77.

22. Adam Smith, *The Theory of Moral Sentiments* (New York: Prometheus Books, 2000), 3.

23. Chan, *A Source Book in Chinese,* 52.

24. Steven Miles, *The Hippocratic Oath and the Ethics of Medicine* (New York: Oxford University Press, 2004); Leon R. Kass, "Is There a Medical Ethics? The Hippocratic Oath and the Sources of Ethical Medicine," in *Toward a More Natural Science: Biology and Human Affairs* (New York: Free Press, 1985).

25. Daniel F. C. Tsai, "Ancient Chinese Medical Ethics and the Four Principles of Biomedical Ethics," *Journal of Medical Ethics* 25:315–21; Daniel F. C. Tsai, "The Bioethical Principles and Confucius' Moral Philosophy," *Journal of Medical Ethics* 31:159–63.

6

Can Justice Be Taught? Valuing Justice and Professionalism in the Medical School Curriculum

Mark G. Kuczewski, Frank Villaume, Heidi Chang, Matthew Fitz, Eva Bading, and Aaron Michelfelder

DOES FOSTERING PROFESSIONALISM ENTAIL A CONCERN FOR JUSTICE?

At first glance, the new emphasis on fostering professionalism in medical students and others in the health-care professions appears to have precious little to do with the concept of justice. Professionalism is often described in terms that focus on the virtues of the individual practitioner and stress the development of personal integrity. Typical issues include self-care, self-presentation, and appropriate interactions with health-care team members and students. In other words, professionalism is often defined in opposition to unprofessional behavior, for example, impairment (e.g., substance abuse); inappropriate dress or tardiness; and abusive behaviors toward residents, medical students, or nurses. These connotations make educating for professionalism a less-than-inspiring endeavor, as it easily becomes about catching outliers on basic measures of habit, custom, and etiquette.

Of course, individual integrity in the professional setting also concerns larger moral issues that involve greater intellectual content. For instance, a variety of potential conflicts of interest present themselves to physicians in their dealings with pharmaceutical companies, insurers, and other commercial organizations with a financial stake in the work of the medical profession.

These issues are sometimes conceptualized as species of justice "writ small" in that they can be regulatory matters for the individual practitioner, the profession, the health-care institution, or the state. But it seems somewhat gratuitous, even grandiose, to employ the term "justice" if that's all that is meant by it. However, it is simple to argue that professionalism entails a concern for justice in larger ways as well. Three considerations are paramount.

First, professions have a contract with society, an explicit and implicit set of duties that entails a conception of justice. Our society underwrites the education and training of physicians in a number of ways, provides tax exemption to nonprofit health-care facilities, and our government is the single largest payer for medical services in the country. In return, a variety of things are expected from the profession, including explicit duties articulated in laws, court decisions, and state and local regulations. But a number of duties are more implicitly contained within institutional practices, such as defining and meeting peer-review standards and standards of care. When social expectations are greater than the reality offered, standards that are left to the profession and to medical institutions, such as assuming a burden of charity care for the poor, are explicitly articulated by the courts and regulators.[1] Clearly, society and the profession are engaged in a debate over what being a profession entails. The demands of social justice, however vague or unarticulated, are at issue in the dialogue. Physicians will do well to have a defined sense of the relationship of professionalism and justice to serve as their moral compass in these waters.

Second, caring for patients likely will raise questions of justice for each individual practitioner. Because academic medical centers treat a large number of uninsured patients,[2] social and public health issues are routinely presented to physicians in training as part of the data of the history and physical. As physicians seek to build a practice, they must make decisions in questions concerning what kinds of insurance they will accept (e.g., Medicaid), where they will practice, and what kind of payer mix is appropriate. The way a physician responds to these questions will implicitly contain responses to the needs of the community and will likely be based on the physician's sense of fairness.

Third, physicians are naturally looked to as leaders by the public and should seek to be worthy of that role. The public seems to understand that our health-care system is under stress and in need of remedies, even if they are suspicious of wholesale changes.[3] It would seem obvious that they might think that physicians have some guidance to offer in this regard. Furthermore, a variety of factors lead to physicians being seen as fairly trustworthy as a group.[4] Of perhaps even greater importance, by virtue of their economic power and educational level, physicians as a group are poised to effect change and are likely to undertake such roles routinely. That is, physicians are likely to try to change things they see as wrong, and their professional organizations tend to have corresponding lobbying agendas. This poses both a danger and an opportunity. The danger is that physicians will reflexively pursue their own interests without giving adequate attention to the interests of the public. For instance, while reforming the malpractice system may be a noble goal, physician organizations have tended to focus their attention on the very narrow goal of capping jury awards and have offered few proposals that seek to compensate the many injured patients who do not pursue legal action or to deal with preventable injuries to patients.[5] As a result, physician groups and organizations may come to be seen merely as special-interest trade organizations rather than professional associations in pursuit of the public good. Of course, there is no reason that physicians who have been trained in a way that nurtures their sense of justice might not seek to advance agendas that serve the interest of the public for whom they care and ask that society foster conditions that aid physicians in caring for them.

We have sought to develop an educational climate that nurtures the development of a sense of justice in our medical students and physicians. To be frank, we are experimenting. We believe that what we are doing is clearly defensible based on the best available evidence. But while the questions of whether virtue and justice can be taught date back to Socrates and Plato, few neat algorithms exist, or are likely to ever exist, for accomplishing these ends. Nevertheless, there is a tradition of virtue theory and education upon which we can draw.[6] As we do so, we shall explain our rationale and experience and remain open to suggestions for improvement. However, I think our approach and design is simple and obvious enough that many schools may already be doing something similar or will desire to do so.

FOSTERING JUSTICE: PHILOSOPHICAL AND PEDAGOGICAL COMMITMENTS

Justice can be a set of theoretical considerations as well as a state of character. As has been suggested from the time of Plato and Aristotle onward, the ideal is for certain concepts or principles of justice to be integrated into the character of a person such that the person has both the desire to act justly and the capacities needed to consider and discern what those actions might be in particular situations.

We could spend much time bogged down in the particulars of what theory of justice should guide us or what principles of justice to make paramount in our educational practices. Our institution has a rich heritage of social justice teachings from the Roman Catholic tradition, particularly that of the sponsoring order known as the Society of Jesus (the Jesuits), from which we draw.[7] While this heritage enriches our environment and permeates the ethos of our faculty and students, one need not accept any particular sectarian or especially controversial views to come to a consensus on some general content that should form the core of a conception of justice in health care at all U.S. medical schools. In many ways, we all know what we are after. The following propositions seem to be relatively uncontroversial except to those who insist on the primacy of narrow personal or special interests.

First, the medical profession must look out for the health of the public. Physicians must be seen as a reliable source of information and as advocates for the promotion of public health and for appropriate care of illness and disease. Second, because the circumstances of people's lives such as poverty, socioeconomic status, ethnicity, and gender can deny persons a fair opportunity for a healthy life or unreasonably limit access to care, the medical profession must consistently call attention to the health and health-care inequities within society and advocate for those most in need. Such a concern has philosophical pedigrees in a variety of philosophical approaches.[8] More recently, we have seen the example of the ubiquitous physician Paul Farmer, who has popularized the Roman Catholic theological construct of the "preferential option for the poor," or "O for the P" as he has dubbed it.[9] As disease and illness clearly prefer the least advantaged in society, physicians must demonstrate a preferential concern for these patients in order to be true to their calling as healers. Furthermore, the medical profession would seem also to have an obligation to foster an awareness of health catastrophes occurring among vulnerable populations around the world. This obligation is partly a concern to promote the health of the U.S. citizenry as the interconnected nature of the contemporary world entails that health problems in one part of the world can easily have a health impact (or economic or security impact) in the rest of the world. But, more importantly, the plight of such unfortunate peoples naturally elicits a response from the virtues of compassion and altruism that characterize physicians. In at least some meager way, humanity is the patient of the medical profession.[10]

In order to produce physicians who have a propensity to act skillfully in accordance with these principles, two assumptions have guided our educational efforts. First, students must perceive that having a sense of justice is valued by their medical school and that this is also prized by the faculty and administrators of the school and the health system within which they train. Second, students need an opportunity to integrate this sense of justice both cognitively and affectively. This entails providing contextual information that coincides with their experiential learning. Furthermore, and perhaps of greater import, educators must provide effective support to students at critical moments when their sense of justice is likely to be undermined. These principles are more or less self-explanatory. However, it is worth considering each carefully so that we might better hit the mark.

WHERE TO START: VALUING
AND INTEGRATING JUSTICE

Valuing justice within the medical school and affiliated health system will reinforce any preexisting propensity that some students possess and will make it more likely that all students will take the topic and related behaviors more seriously. While this may seem a most obvious point, it is one that has been getting lost in the frenzy to evaluate outcomes. That is, evaluating and assessing professionalism are seen as very important. Evaluation is often seen as the same as valuing. "We improve what we measure" has become the mantra of the current era. While this may be true, evaluation is only one way to value behavior and character, and, depending on the method, can be a fairly trivial one.[11] For instance, measurements of personal qualities and behaviors involved in professionalism are sometimes assessed via checklists and can seem to lack meaning and context to students and their evaluators despite being "scientific" in terms of inter-rater reliability. Thus, it is important to have many ways in which the value placed on justice is elaborated. It is not an exaggeration to say that the primary evaluation must be of the institution itself, which should be graded on how it demonstrates the premium it places upon these dimensions of the student.

How do we demonstrate that we value justice as part of medical professionalism at the Stritch School of Medicine? In general, the role modeling of important persons in required portions of the curriculum provides an important clue. Our faculty and health-system administrators have developed a required course called "Business, Professionalism, and Justice" (BPnJ) that explicitly connects justice and professionalism. This course provides a variety of didactic sessions and interactive activities in which the business of medicine is explored in its macroeconomic and microeconomic aspects. The business of medicine is laid out so that the implications for justice of various choices can become transparent. Students are asked to consider what the obligations of the medical profession to advocate for change might be given these current situations.

While there is much that we can say about the cognitive needs that are met through this course, for the present purpose the most important thing to note is that the course shows that our institution values these concerns by 1) requiring the course, and 2) resourcing the course with its best, brightest, and most prestigious faculty members and administrators. While many schools may require important and well-meaning courses but staff them with a small group of specialized faculty, the BPnJ course has lecturers and small-group moderators that include the chief executive officer and a number of senior vice presidents of the health system, the dean of the school of medicine, and a number of department chairs and senior clinicians drawn from a broad array of clinical departments. In this course, the clinical faculty members have the opportunity to explain their responsibilities as administrators and the challenges they confront. As a result, the course is popular and seen as important by the students. Their evaluative comments commonly express the wish that they had had an opportunity to hear these faculty and administrators teach in other venues during their education.

Similarly, the efforts of the students to show excellence in justice and professionalism must be respected, honored, and reinforced (i.e., valued). We have created the honors program in bioethics and professionalism to accomplish these purposes. It is an effort-based program in which students self-identify as wishing to participate and qualify by keeping a portfolio of reflections on relevant activities over three years, and then developing an academic capstone project (i.e., a poster or paper presentation) on one of their activities. They are honored at graduation. Their participation in this program is also noted in their medical school performance evaluation (i.e., "dean's letter") and on their transcript.

The design of the program is meant to provide the message that professionalism, especially its aspects concerning justice, is a worthwhile area of endeavor and research. As an effort-based program, it holds that excellence in this area is available to those who make the necessary investment of their intellectual and personal resources, including their time. (Approximately one-third of our students participate in this program.) Furthermore, participants are mentored through the program by faculty mentors of their choosing. The participation of these mentors, some of whom are recruited at the request of the students, values the activity through role modeling. But more importantly, the mentor is available to support the student and assist in intellectual integration of the lessons at important developmental moments. Let us see how this works by examining sample student reflections.

REINFORCING AND SUPPORTING JUSTICE
THROUGH REFLECTION

Reflections of Mike O'Reilly
(second-year medical student)

STUDENT GOAL

I have been involved with community health this year, with a goal of attending one clinic session per month. My goal for this event is to continue to develop my relationship and communication skills with patients, and in particular those patients that are of different socioeconomic backgrounds. I feel that this is a valuable goal because one's background can be revealing as to [a patient's] insight into [his or her] illness . . . [and] ability to recover and maintain good health and can allow me to better understand the perspectives of patients in general. I also feel that it will be a positive way to contribute to society, offering whatever medical services I can for four to five hours a month. This event will continually challenge my communication skills as I attempt to bridge the gap between me and primarily Spanish-speaking patients.

REFLECTION ON ACTIVITY

After one semester volunteering at community health, I feel like I have had a positive experience overall. My interviewing skills have been improved and become more focused, and my Spanish has become somewhat easier to use despite only using it once a month.

Perhaps the most beneficial experiences I have had from community health have been the interesting patient encounters that have taken place while I have been there. On any given night I will usually see two patients in a four to five hour span. I am still surprised at how long it takes to interview patients (especially in Spanish), perform the necessary physical exam steps, and present the case to a third- or fourth-year student and eventually to an attending working at the clinic, each of whom need to ask their own questions and review the findings I have given them. I would estimate that most patients spend three hours at least, from arriving at the clinic until they leave with their medicine. The reason that most of the patients come to community health is that they have no health insurance and are aware of a new or continuing medical condition that they feel they can take a large amount of time out of their schedule to have examined. I feel that it is unfair to them to have to wait so long, just because of their socioeconomic status, and to find that they will be confronted with a barrage of medical students who are essentially practicing their medical skills (under supervision, of course). While it is an excellent learning tool for the students, and a way for the attending physicians to give back to the community, I find myself embarrassed by my lack of knowledge and constantly asking patients to wait until we can all figure out what we are doing. Perhaps this situation is the same at hospitals like Loyola, but I am not yet familiar enough with the role of the students there to compare.

On the other hand, another observation that has surprised me is the gratitude that the patients express toward the medical students for whatever we can do to help. It has been a good lesson to learn . . . that even just the small acts of asking questions and running around looking up information and refilling prescriptions can go a long way toward making a patient satisfied with the care they are receiving. After forgetting certain steps of the physical exam and having a patient take off his shoes and socks for the third time, I overheard the patient say to my translator that he was "just happy that somebody is so concerned about his health." It made me question just what kind of care this patient had received in the past, because I know that my care, although thorough, was far from efficient and easy. It has truly been a lesson in how to appreciate the way of life of others who are less fortunate and has made me more aware.

One final point that I have been questioning is the role of the medical industry in the lives of the economically disadvantaged. A story to illustrate [this] was one night when a patient diagnosed with rheumatoid arthritis needed a refill of her prescription nonsteroidal anti-inflammatory medication (NSAID). This is a drug that is donated by the drug company to our clinic, but for people who have health insurance, the company charges about eight dollars per day for one dose. When I presented the patient to one of the attending physicians, he immediately switched her to ibuprofen, a drug that requires more dosing and has more side effects that the patient complained of from past experiences but is far cheaper and can be provided by the county for the rest of the patient's life. When I objected to giving her a drug that was inferior to one that we had a healthy supply of, the physician asked me to consider whether it is fair for a "poor person" to receive this drug, when many other people who can actually afford it are denied it by their insurance companies. He proceeded to tell her to lose weight and take the ibupro-fen with a meal to reduce the irritating side effects. The idea of rationing medical resources was one that I had heard of but never experienced in person, and I was asked to send her off with the ibuprofen medication instead of the better drug. I feel that in this situation we should have given her the best drugs that we had, and as for the millions of people who suffer from arthritis, I still feel that it is fair to give them the most effective drugs for their individual condition. But I learned in an unpleas-ant way from this physician that the poor are truly disadvantaged, regardless of whether they can come to our clinic. In a way, it was the way that this physician treated her that made her situation even worse. I suspect that I will be reflecting on this issue much more in the future.

Advisor Comments

Your reflection on your work at community health is very good. You brought up some substantive points on several dimensions, e.g., the atti-tudes of those you treat, the subtle unfairness of the system, etc. This is excellent. Keep up the good work.

You might consider in the future what you think the response of the medical profession to these situations ought to be. You might also con-sider analyzing the issue of the NSAID versus ibuprofen at greater length with the physician or in regard to some other patient in the future. That is, which medication is best can be a complicated issue, e.g., which medication is best in the abstract versus which is best for this patient given a variety of circumstances. It is an issue that would make a worthy capstone project.

This reflection shows several themes that are often seen in student reflections. First, student motivations in providing service are often multilayered. That is, the goal of service and care of the disadvantaged may be primary but is also supported by the desire for hands-on clinical experience, experience that is initially easier to come by early in volunteer settings rather than in school. The related themes of feeling inadequate to assist in care and learning that sheer attention and concern for the patient, in fact, are worthwhile offerings. The patient as teacher and the student as caregiver in a broad sense permeate many students' writings.

This reflective exercise provides an opportunity for the student to own these important discoveries in his development and to highlight these lessons as part of who he is becoming. Clearly, this advisor sees the primary task as reinforcement of these noble inclinations and the continued encouragement of the process of self-discovery. The reflection also contains systemic issues concerning the appropriate medication to be prescribed to the patient. Written before recent revelations concerning attendant risks of various NSAIDs, it raises the question of whether all departures from the standard of care are unjust simpliciter and to be resisted by the physician, or whether there are some treatments that may be better for the disadvantaged patient based on considerations such as sustainability. Because the reflection is rich from the point of view of the student's understanding of the caregiver-patient relationship, the advisor chose not to risk sidetracking the focus by taking up this complicated issue of appropriate treatment but simply to mark its potential for further investigation. Nevertheless, identifying it as such calls to the attention of the student that points of frustration with the system are worthy of exploration and need not simply end in frustration and disillusionment.

Reflections of Vera Parisi (second-year medical student)

STUDENT GOAL

This trip to Haiti will provide me with a wonderful opportunity to gain experience with service work in the third world. I hope to gain clinical experience as well as improve my ability to work with others in potentially stressful conditions. I hope to learn about the delivery of culturally sensitive medicine and tailor my interactions with patients to reflect their values, beliefs, concerns, and interests. As doing medical work in underserved populations has always been a motivating factor in my desire to become a physician, I look forward to getting a taste of the struggles and potentials for such service work.

REFLECTION ON ACTIVITY

This past summer I spent ten days in Haiti with a group from Stritch School of Medicine. Since I have limited clinical skills I spent my days in the clinic learning and observing, doing whatever small tasks I could.

My feelings while in Haiti spanned a wide gamut. I was saddened by the poverty, by the number of unmet needs of so many people. My stomach leapt to my throat [when I saw] the many malnourished and starving people. It's a terrible injustice that there's enough food to feed the world, but rich countries, like ours, pay farmers to let crops rot in storehouses to keep prices up. When one considers the number of people we saw suffering in a small amount of time, and in a small country, it's mind numbing to think of the sheer number of people in like circumstance around the world.

I felt guilty and ashamed: guilty for having so much while others have so little, and ashamed by the sense of entitlement pervasive in American culture. We have done little to warrant our wealth, it was simply good fortune that we were born in the U.S. and not ninety miles south in Haiti. I also felt ashamed by the realization that the people in Haiti have so little because we have so much. And while the unequal distribution of wealth saddens me, the question becomes, what am I willing to do about it? Am I really willing to live more modestly so that others could live more decently? My presence in Haiti did not soothe my conscience, rather it served to make me feel more guilty. A medical student, without any skills to help the people, taxing Haiti's already limited resources. Although we brought much needed and appreciated medical supplies we really contributed little else to the people of Haiti. I probably could have done more for the people if I simply wrote out my $500 check to the Saint Boniface Haiti Foundation and stayed at home.

My time in Haiti also made me question my faith, and question why God would allow such suffering to persist. I believe that God is love and that He is all powerful. Holding babies, orphans, who were so emaciated just made me question, why. Why would He allow this to go on? And since most of the people we met doing amazing service work in Haiti were Catholic I wonder how they have settled this question of why in their own hearts.

The medical work in Haiti made me reexamine my choice to become a physician. Through my training in public health I realized that although a career in public health would allow me to help people, I would sorely miss the opportunity to work with patients and to develop relationships with the people I was trying to help. But while in Haiti I felt that our medical care was simply applying band-aids. We treated symptoms of an underlying disease. Haiti needs infrastructure, clean water, food, and the ability to meet the very basic needs of her people. While providing medical care is necessary, and it's making a difference to the patient in front of you, it's not addressing the causes, it's not making a long-term real difference. Which brought me back to why I went into public health initially: time spent in the ER, applying band-aids, very similar to the feeling I had in the hospital in Haiti.

I'm not sure how my experience in Haiti will impact my future, be it professional or personal. Since coming back from Haiti the words of a James Taylor song often spring into my head: "Every now and then the things I lean on lose their meaning . . . and I find myself careening into places where I should not let me go." I guess the new challenge is how to keep the experience from making me pessimistic and completely disillusioned about the potential for change, and the possibility of making a positive difference.

ADVISOR COMMENTS

I struggle with this over and over and over again. Make it a point to go back to Fr. Mark's orphanage at some point in your life if you can. Take on a project, even if smaller in scope. When I went back to Nigeria and witnessed the growth, it renewed my faith . . . my purpose. Eight Daughters of Charity . . . making it happen in a poor country where the retarded and crippled are left to die. You will have skills one day . . . skills that will take you wherever and allow you to do whatever. When I am tired of fighting with the administration here, I remind myself of Fr. Mark or the Daughters.

Vera Parisi's reflection shows some of the same themes as those of Mike O'Reilly, albeit on a much grander scale. For instance, while Mike O'Reilly was frustrated with the health-care system because it restricted access to state-of-the-art medications, Vera Parisi is frustrated with the health-care system on a global scale. This frustration seems to boil over into despair that one human being, even a physician with public health training, can make any significant difference in the lives of the least advantaged. She finds herself challenged at a personal level, feeling shame at her own privileged station in life and her lack of efficacy. This naturally goes beyond self-doubt to a more profound spiritual doubt about her God. She wonders how other religious persons make sense of these matters.

Her advisor responds to this invitation by relating that he struggles with these matters as well and tries to offer an example to balance her despair with a single example of hope. Of interest is that he seems to indicate that these moments of frustration in the face of systemic injustice are not confined to experiences in the developing world but present themselves at home in the clinical setting as well.

We cannot know how effective the consolation the advisor offers is. However, we can once again note that the portfolio has provided the student an opportunity to express her concerns and spiritual state of affairs rather than keep them to herself. Furthermore, this reflection and the response of her advisor are moments early in the three-year process of developing the honors portfolio. This interaction provides one basis for future interaction. As a result, there is someone to respond in word and example as this student continues to confront these challenges.

THE ELEMENTS OF TEACHING JUSTICE: DOING, REFLECTING, CONTEXTUALIZING

In sum, we see that teaching justice (i.e., fostering a sense of justice and a propensity to act in accordance with this sense) requires certain things on the part of the student and certain things on the part of his or her learning environment (the medical school and health system).

As Aristotle noted, becoming virtuous requires doing virtuous actions. One can then understand the reasons for such actions. One's discernment of the particulars of good action can be improved through such practical philosophizing, and we can become inclined to better "hit the mark" in doing virtuous things.[12] As a result, our approach to fostering justice requires

1. Doing (Activity)
2. Reflecting
3. Contextualizing

The students do certain activities and reflect on them, and we assist in cognitive consideration of the systemic context of these activities through mentor feedback and the Business, Professionalism, and Justice curriculum. We are rather assured that this framework is the proper one to bring about the desired outcome—just physicians. However, we are continually attempting to find and refine the means for implementing this framework. For instance, we recently implemented a required reflection exercise on a modest service activity in our first-year physician-patient relationship course, which is called "Patient-Centered Medicine-1" (PCM-1). This is meant to introduce all our first-year students to the justice aspect of professionalism in medicine before we offer them an opportunity to enroll in the honors program. We plan to provide an opportunity to revisit these reflections in the fourth-year BPnJ course in future years, and thereby for each student to further understand his or her moral and cognitive development.

This virtue approach to justice and professionalism not only imposes requirements on the student but also on the community in which the learner learns. The medical school and health system(s) in which the students train must explicitly and implicitly value justice and must provide mechanisms of support to students when they are at critical junctures in their development. We have outlined how this is done explicitly by the required curriculum and honoring student effort through the honors program. It is implicitly valued through the role modeling of the high-level faculty members and administrators who participate in the professionalism and honors curricula. And, of course, we looked at the support and coaching provided in the mentoring provided to honors program students.

What should also be obvious is that when approximately one-third of all students are engaged in the honors program, it leavens the entire environment and adds to the sense of the environment as one that values justice and professionalism. In this way, our programming is a self-fulfilling prophecy.[13]

NOTES

We wish to acknowledge the American Medical Association's Strategies in Teaching and Evaluating Professionalism project (AMA STEP), whose support has contributed to this work.

1. S. Baksh, "Non-profit Hospitals Face More Questions," *Washington Times,* May 27, 2005; M. Schlesinger, S. Mitchell, and B. H. Gray, "Public Expectations of Nonprofit and For-Profit Ownership in American Medicine: Clarifications and Implications," *Health Affairs* 23 (6): 181–91.

2. M. Lewin and S. Altman, eds., *America's Health Care Safety Net: Intact but Endangered* (Washington, DC: National Academy Press, 2000), 42–44.

3. R. J. Blendon, M. Brodie, D. E. Altman, J. M. Benson, and E. C. Hamel, "Voters and Health Care in the 2004 Election," *Health Affairs* Web Exclusive, March 1, 2005.

4. D. W. Moore, "Nurses Top List in Honesty and Ethics Poll," Gallup Organization, December 7, 2004, www.gallup.com/poll/content/login.aspx?ci = 14236 (accessed June 6, 2005).

5. M. J. Mehlman, "Malpractice Reforms: Are They Fair?" *Clinics in Perinatology* 32 (1): 235–49; R. R. Bovbjerg, "Malpractice Crisis and Reform," *Clinics in Perinatology* 32 (1): 203–33.

6. A. MacIntyre, *After Virtue* (Indiana: University of Notre Dame Press, 1981); E. Pellegrino and D. Thomasma, *The Virtues in Medical Practice* (New York: Oxford University Press, 1993).

7. M. Kuczewski, E. Bading, M. Langbein, and B. Henry, "Fostering Professionalism: The Loyola Model," *Cambridge Quarterly of Healthcare Ethics,* 12 (2):161–66.

8. J. Rawls, *A Theory of Justice* (Cambridge, MA: Harvard University Press, 1971); T. Kidder, *Mountains beyond Mountains* (New York: Random House, 2003); C. E. Curran, *Catholic Social Teaching, 1891–Present* (Washington, DC: Georgetown University Press, 2002).

9. Kidder, *Mountains beyond Mountains*; C. E. Curran, *Catholic Social Teaching, 1891–Present* (Washington, DC: Georgetown University Press, 2002); see especially "Part One: The Social Responsibility of Catholic Health Care Services," from the United States Conference of Catholic Bishops, *Ethical and Religious Directives for Catholic Health Care Services, 4th edition* (Washington, DC: 2001).

10. Medical Professionalism Project, "'Medical Professionalism in the New Millennium: A Physician Charter,'" *Annals of Internal Medicine* 136 (2002): 243–46.

11. D. T. Stern, A. Wojtczak, and M. R. Schwarz, "IIME Task Force for Assessment: The Assessment of Global Minimum Essential Requirements in Medical Education," *Medical Teacher* 25 (6): 589–95.

12. Aristotle, *The Nicomachean Ethics,* book 2, 4–6. Terence Irwin, trans., Indianapolis, IN: Hackett Publishing Company, 2000.

13. Furthermore, these efforts are resulting in a certain satisfaction among our students. Our evaluation data show that our students far exceed national averages in feeling confident that they have been well prepared in professionalism, health economics, and health systems.

7

Initiating and Evaluating a Program in Ethics and Professionalism for Medical Residents

Eugene V. Boisaubin, Virginia Greene,
Allison R. Ownby, and Mark Farnie

The University of Texas Medical School at Houston, one of five medical schools in the University of Texas system, is located in the Texas Medical Center, the world's largest health complex, in Houston, Texas. The Department of Medicine Residency Program, within the school of medicine, is large, with over one hundred fifty residents dispersed over three years of training and all working toward board certification in internal medicine. There is one senior and two associate program directors of the residency, who are responsible for the training of the residents, as well as the departmental chairman. The American Board of Internal Medicine, which certifies all internal medicine trainees, as well as the Accreditation Council for Graduate Medical Education (ACGME) and its Residency Review Committee (RRC) have required that all graduate trainees demonstrate a number of clinical competencies, including ethical behavior and professionalism.[1] But what needs to be taught in this curriculum has been only generally alluded to by the accrediting groups.[2] Even more difficult has been the challenge to identify and utilize effective means of evaluation for appropriate ethical and professional knowledge and behaviors.[3] Obviously, there is also a broader societal obligation to teach physicians of the future how to practice not only competent but compassionate and professionally acceptable medicine.

Approximately three years ago, a curriculum in ethics and professionalism (E&P) was started, primarily as a series of noontime lectures to teach residents the fundamental concepts and practices of these disciplines. Initially, there was no formal evaluation system of the resulting knowledge or behaviors regarding E&P. However, over the past two years, a more comprehensive program to not only educate but also evaluate residents in training has been instituted, and this chapter describes its evolution and impact.

THE EDUCATIONAL MODALITIES

The educational modalities utilized in teaching the E&P curriculum are primarily based upon traditional approaches used to train graduate-level residents. The residents and the faculty are familiar with these traditional formats, which include the following: noontime medical conferences, "morning report," and the Clinical Pathologic Conference (CPC). In addition, since the number of hours available to teach residents has been effectively reduced through the stringently applied work-hour limitation rules, teaching time has to be used extremely efficiently. Since there is good pedagogical evidence that adults learn through a variety of educational means, which include real situations that will be encountered in both training and practice, the curriculum is designed to present a spectrum of learning opportunities, utilizing 'real-life' scenarios for the resident as much as possible. The learning modalities used primarily in this curriculum are the following:

Large Group Learning (LGL) Sessions

This modality is based upon the traditional noontime medical conference with a lecture-hall format and is organized with a faculty speaker with lecture content created around a theme topic. However, unlike a purely traditional lecture, the speaker introduces the presentation theme with a brief clinical vignette, and then additional vignettes are given before each subsection of the topic. For example, a session on advance directives might begin with a vignette in which a patient expresses his or her interest in completing one of these documents, and the speaker would then ask the residents how they would respond. Later vignettes would include an advance directive example in which the written guidelines are unfortunately ambiguous, and a final vignette could reflect a scenario in which the patient who has completed a directive is now incompetent, but the family challenges the validity of the guidelines. The residents in attendance are asked to respond as to how they would approach each vignette, and a brief discussion ensues. By the end of the lecture hour, the overall theme has been addressed through these several vignettes, the resulting discussion, and summary points made by the presenter. These sessions are integrated into the typical daily lecture series that all residents are required to attend, and usually one session is offered every month. These sessions form the didactic backbone of the E&P curriculum and cover a variety of essential themes that are delivered over an academic year's time. The typical LGL topics that are presented annually are listed in table 7.1.

E&P Morning Report

For decades, "Morning Report" has been a classic academic teaching modality in which residents present cases to their peers and faculty in what is typically an hour-long session, held daily on five or six days out of seven. The presented cases are traditionally selected from recently admitted hospital cases and are chosen because of their immediate diagnostic or therapeutic interest or challenge. With the E&P Report, usually held one or two times a month, patient-based cases with challenging problems in ethics and/or professionalism, rather than traditional organ pathology, are presented and an educational dialogue ensues among the case presenter, the audience, and an E&P faculty educator. Typical case scenarios include a patient who refuses recommended medical care, or a question of confidentiality involving the family members of a patient with AIDS. These case discussions can not be planned ahead but instead reflect the more spontaneous educational needs of the residents, and their timeliness and "need to learn" quality can make them powerful educational experiences. In addition, because they represent ongo

Table 7.1.   Core Large Group Learning Session Topics in the E&P Curriculum

E&P Dilemmas in Emergency Care

Introduction to Ethical Issues in End-of-Life Care

Advance Planning in End-of-Life Care: Advance Directives and Do Not Resuscitate (DNR)

Dilemmas in Consent and Determining Patient Competency

Defining Brain Death and the Persistent Vegetative State (PVS)

Issues in Patient Confidentiality and Institutional Guidelines (HIPAA)

E&P Issues in the Care of the AIDS Patient

Boundary Issues in the Patient-Physician Relationship

Addressing and Preventing Medical Error

Conflicts of Interest in Training and Practice

Special Patient Dilemmas: The Jehovah's Witness

Identifying and Treating the Impaired Physician

Treating and Preventing Physician Stress and Burnout

ing, real-time, problematic clinical cases in the hospital faced by the residents, the discussion and conclusions provide valuable assistance to the physician in training who is trying to learn how to provide both competent and compassionate care.

Clinical Pathologic Conference (CPC)

This is one of the most traditional of educational conferences in medical and surgical training and focuses on the analysis and discussion of the postmortem case of a patient who has recently died. This particular modality is presented in a lecture format by an E&P faculty member. The uniqueness of the E&P CPC is that the deceased patient's case reflects a dilemma or controversy in E&P, rather than only the traditional issues of differential diagnosis and/or treatment. For example, almost any patient's death, particularly after a long illness, inherently raises ethical issues of when decisions to limit further treatment might have been made before the patient's death. Also possibly germane might be issues of the real or potential benefit of an advance directive to help better define when and what treatment might have been limited. Real or potential conflict between health-care members and the patient and/or family, or among caregivers themselves, might also have occurred and hindered optimal medical management and care. In essence, almost the entire spectrum of ethical and professional challenges that compose "end-of-life" care can be addressed in these sessions. Last, it is not uncommon that minor or major errors have occurred at some point in the care trajectory and need to be openly discussed. Addressing medical error is a very important element in medical professionalism, and few residents have been instructed adequately in terms of how to address these issues among themselves and their faculty, or how honest they should be when patients or family members ask about unexpected outcomes.[4]

Program for Physician Well-Being

Physicians in training and practice cannot fully treat the psychosocial needs of their patients unless their own needs concerning both ethical and personal values have been adequately addressed. Problems such as depression, marital discord, substance abuse, and even financial stressors can detract from the resident's ability to gain appropriate balance between his or her personal and professional life. And when these problems are significant, they can easily 'spill over' into the professional role and compromise performance and even patient care. When present, therefore, these problems need to be identified and addressed early on so that they do not adversely affect the personal and professional life. Beginning two years ago, the school of medicine established a program with the university's Employee Assistance Program to offer free counseling to resident physicians for a variety of problems or concerns, including financial, marital, and child-rearing issues. Also available is a program for physician impairment, including substance abuse and psychiatric disorders. Resident physicians may refer themselves or may be referred by the program directors if the problem is affecting their professional role. True impairment is usually treated in an outpatient setting with a binding contract signed by the resident and program directors that assures the needed treatment, follow-up, and monitoring and addresses the possibility of relapse.[5]

Last, although neither part of the formal curriculum nor directly under the control of the Department of Medicine, is the Ethics Consultation Service, which is an extension of the hospital ethics committee and is offered throughout the main teaching facility of the residency program, Memorial Hermann Hospital. With this program, the ethics consultant on call answers all consultation requests initiated by the physicians, nurses, or other health-care professionals in the hospital. More than 65 percent of the consultations involve end-of-life care questions. The consultant may be able to resolve the dilemma by simply providing needed information or by clarifying a hospital policy, but in cases where a formal complete consultation is required, additional committee members may be involved. The great majority of the ethics consultations involve services with residents in training, so there is the very real inclusion of an educational component with each consultation that involves house officers.

Evaluating the Educational Program and the Residents

Many, if not all, internal medicine residency programs have some kind of elementary curriculum in biomedical ethics, and a few in professionalism, although having a comprehensive program with multiple distinct modalities for education, as described above, is unusual. Even more unusual is an internal medicine residency program that has a comprehensive evaluation program that attempts to measure a resident's acquisition of the requisite knowledge, skills, and behavior in ethics and professionalism. The E&P curriculum currently has four modalities in place to measure these qualities and behaviors. The results of these measurements are placed into a E&P folder in a resident's permanent record.

Traditional RRC Evaluation Methods

Required of all accredited programs in internal medicine is a formal, biannual face-to-face evaluation of all components of the resident's performance, including professionalism. This evaluation is derived primarily from performance reports completed monthly by the supervising attending physicians. The evaluation sessions are conducted by the program directors, all performance data is reviewed, and recommendations for improvement or change are made and documented in the resident's permanent record. Included now in this evaluation is a review of the content of the E&P folder.

Self-Appraisal

As part of the required evaluation sessions with each resident, the program directors complete a page-long form that rates the resident's performance on a five-point Likert scale based upon fourteen different criteria, including issues of professionalism. Just prior to the face-to-face meeting, the residents are asked to complete an identical form in which they evaluate themselves. Therefore, the first part of the evaluation involves comparing the resident's self-evaluation with that of the program directors'. Typically, the resident's evaluation rates him- or herself the same as, or one point lower than, that of the director. The somewhat lower average probably reflects modesty, or the commonly accepted social caveat that one shouldn't rate oneself too highly in front of evaluating superiors. But two other patterns may be observed and are cause for reflection and even concern. First is the resident who evaluates herself much lower than the director and may suffer from low self-esteem, possibly as part of underlying clinical depression, and may need referral to the physician well-being program. Second, the resident who evaluates him- or herself very highly, when there are clear areas of documented deficiency, may not have adequate insight into his or her limitations and may need additional counseling from the director, and even psychological therapy.

Peer Evaluation

Related to, but different in important ways from, self-review is peer review. Once annually, all second- and third-year residents are asked to complete an anonymous form that evaluates their peers on a variety of professional scales, including integrity, altruism and willingness to assume responsibility. Since the program is large, residents are asked not to comment upon other residents with whom they have not worked. When completed, each resident receives a numerical scorecard with his or her individual marks and a comparison to the group average. These reports also are added to the resident's professionalism file.

Standardized Patient Evaluation Program

An additional and particularly innovative evaluation method is the unannounced Standardized Patient Evaluation Program (SPEP). This evaluation tool has been used in the residency program for the past three years, in collaboration with the Office of Educational Programs. The program provides a method by which targeted residents are observed and evaluated on their professionalism skills, in addition to their medical knowledge, by an unannounced standardized patient posing as a new patient with medical problems. The use of standardized patients (SP) has been a staple of medical education and evaluation throughout student and resident training programs in America for over a decade.[6] The SPEP begins with the SP, a trained lay person scripted with a specific illness or complaint who presents to a specifically assigned resident in his or her half-day-a-week continuity clinic for a prearranged appointment as a new, or "real," patient. The resident does not know that the patient is not genuine, although residents have been told that they will encounter an unannounced SP as part of their evaluation process in the course of their clinic experience. The patient is also thought to be "real" by everyone at the clinic except for the clinic manager, the clinic staff member who scheduled the appointment, and the attending physician, who is notified that the evaluation will be occurring. However, the attending has no role in the evaluation process. In fact, it is preferred that the attending is not involved, since residents might change the quality of their evaluation if they know they are being observed. The SP evaluates the resident on his or her professional behavior and communication skills, as well as medical knowledge and clinical examination skills. Even at the end of the encounter, the SP does not identify him- or herself nor provide immediate feedback to the resident, but he or she later completes a written evaluation of the encounter, including a report on the resident's professional attitudes and behavior, as well as a scoring of the correct components of both the history and physical examination. Additional general feedback is provided during a postexam follow-up session with all the residents being tested, the program directors, and a member of the Office of Educational Programs. At that meeting all residents receive their individual evaluations as well as blinded numerical comparisons with their peers. The individual and comparison scores are added to the permanent folder of each participating resident and are rereviewed at the time of the semiannual evaluation, during which time corrective action might be recommended for residents with low scores.

Although an evaluation of every resident would be ideal, the large size of the residency program makes this impossible, since it would require large numbers of trained SPs, with their attendant costs, and extensive administrative time and energy. Therefore, a total of twelve to fifteen second-year residents are selected annually to participate in the program. Residents who are selected include those brand new to the program and those who have been perceived by the program directors as having possible deficiencies in performance, particularly in professionalism, as noted by evaluators in the past year. In addition, a randomly selected number of "control" residents from the second year are chosen whose previous evaluations have indicated competent professional performance to date. A variety of illness scripts and clinical scenarios are used each year for the residents, since it is important they do not "catch on" to the trained patients and or tell their colleagues that, for example, the "patient with headache and a quirky medical history" is not a real patient. This year the program will offer the residents who perform below a competent level of performance an individualized learning plan designed to improve their skills. These same residents will be reassessed in the spring with another unannounced patient visit to determine if any improvement or change in their skills has occurred.

The data have been both well received and occasionally challenged. Most of the residents have appreciated the opportunity to have been involved in the program, and many of them said they thought resources should be allocated to allow every second-year resident to have an SP experience.

Medical Student Evaluation of Residents

The most recently employed evaluation system utilizes medical students rotating through the department on their core clinical rotations. The clinical students evaluate both their supervising first-year residents (interns) and senior residents on the team to which they are assigned. At the end of the clinical rotation, each student is asked to anonymously complete an evaluation of the residents' professionalism, including their attitude toward patients, willingness and ability to work with and teach the students, and the residents' integrity and respect for the privacy and confidentiality of the patients. These comments are recorded on an evaluation form with a Likert scale for each professional behavior, and a space is provided for written comments at the bottom. Much of the data received regarding the residents are positive and complimentary, but occasionally a student gives a low score to a resident or provides comments about a resident that suggest behavior that must be addressed and remediated.

In summary, the E&P Program now provides both a comprehensive curriculum in medical ethics and professionalism and an extensive, or "360-degree," view of the attitudes and behaviors of the residents, as captured by the four evaluation modalities.[7] Two other methods of "360-degree" resident evaluation, ratings by nurses and by patients and their families, have been attempted by others but not utilized by our program. First, we have found the turnover in nurse positions and the frequent rotation changes by our residents as they move through three hospitals in our institution have made it difficult for them to adequately evaluate each resident. However, negative behaviors or attitudes of major concern, as exhibited by a resident, are recorded in 'incident reports' from the nursing staff, which are sent to the program directors and may result in an immediate face-to-face meeting with the offending resident. Second, we have found patient and/or family evaluations not to be of great help, since the care recipients have difficulty telling one resident, or even medical students, from each other, and because they tend to give generally positive and uncritical evaluations to all physicians involved in their care. An important observation made by the program directors is that in the great majority of cases in which a resident is critically identified by one of the above evaluation techniques, they have already been identified as having a potential problem by another previous evaluation. This gives credence to the entire program and suggests that rather than "catching" a good resident in a rare, unprotected moment of bad behavior, we are identifying residents who demonstrate repetitive behavior problems and are clearly in need of assistance. This also makes the job of the program directors easier when it comes to the biannual face-to-face evaluation, because it is more difficult for a resident to deny that a problem is present when several different evaluations by different people in differing settings have been collected.

NOTES

1. American Board of Internal Medicine, *Project Professionalism,* Philadephia: American Board of Internal Medicine 2001, 1–41; Accreditation Council for Graduate Medical Education, www.acgme.org.

2. American Board of Internal Medicine, *Project Professionalism.*

3. E. L. Arnold, L. L. Blank, K. E. Race, and N. Cipparrone, "Can Professionalism Be Measured? The Development of a Scale for Use in the Medical Environment," *Academic Medicine* 78 (10): 1119–21; L. Arnold, "Assessing Professional Behavior: Yesterday, Today and Tomorrow," *Academic Medicine* 77 (6): 502–15.

4. T. Gallagher, A. Waterman, A. Ebers, V. Fraser, and W. Levinson, "Patients' and Physicians' Attitudes Regarding the Disclosure of Medical Errors," *Journal of the American Medical Association* 289 (2003): 1001–7.

5. E. Boisaubin and R. Levine, "Identifying and Assisting the Impaired Physician," *American Journal of Medical Sciences* 322 (2001): 31–36.

6. M. D. Prislin, D. Lie, J. Shapiro, J. Boker, and S. Radecki, "Using Standardized

Patients to Assess Medical Students' Professionalism," *Academic Medicine* 76 (10): 90–92.

7. E. A. Hesketh, F. Anderson, G. M. Bagnall, C. P. Driver, D. A. Johnston, D. Marshall, J. Needham, G. Orr, and K. Walker, "Using a 360 Degree Diagnostic Screening Tool to Provide an Evidence Trail of Junior Doctor Performance throughout Their First Postgraduate Year," *Medical Teacher* 27 (2005): 219–33.

8

Two Faces of Professionalism

DeWitt C. Baldwin Jr.

"Virtue? Can it be taught? Or how does it come? Do I know that? So far from knowing whether it can be taught or can't be taught . . . I don't even know what virtue is."[1]

A PROBLEM WITH DEFINITIONS

From the beginning of its meteoric rise in interest among medical leaders and educators, the term "professionalism" has posed major problems in definition and assessment. As with many other value-oriented ideologically based constructs, such as humanism, morality, and spirituality, most people seem to have little problem recognizing it when they see it, or fail to see it but seem to have a great deal of difficulty deciding precisely what it is and how to teach or transmit it to others.

Some time ago, I assembled an alphabetized list of fifty-two different attributes or descriptive qualities, such as altruism, empathy, service, responsibility, compassion, and integrity, that are commonly associated with, or gleaned from, the respective literatures of professionalism, humanism, morality, and spirituality. I then asked a group of colleagues to assign each attribute or quality to as many of these four constructs as seemed appropriate. Their responses showed that there was an extremely high degree of overlap among the attributes and qualities assigned to these highly value-oriented constructs. Eighteen, or 35 percent, of the listed attributes ended up being assigned to all four constructs, while another sixteen (31 percent) were ascribed to as many as three of them. Furthermore, while the highest percentage of overlap was between professionalism and humanism (65 percent), there also was a 62-percent overlap in attributes between professionalism and morality, and a 46-percent overlap with spirituality.[2]

This sort of confusion has posed problems for many students, trainees, and younger physicians, as well as for the medical educators who attempt to teach professionalism. How can a particular quality that is so important and highly regarded be learned and successfully attained if it cannot be defined and measured with the precision expected of the rest of science and education? Medical students are extremely adept at absorbing mountains of information if they know what it is and where to look for it. But so far, this important topic must seem to them highly amorphous and elusive. What we obviously long for is the certainty expressed by Humpty Dumpty to Alice in Lewis Carroll's *Through the Looking Glass*: "When *I* use a word, it means just what I choose it to mean—neither more nor less."[3]

The first two articles in a recent issue of the *American Journal of Bioethics* appear to illustrate this problem. In the first, Wear and Kuczewski address the phenomenon of professionalism's rising presence and place in the field and in the literature, thankfully calling for the need to pause and reflect further on this subject before it proceeds down the path of unqualified acceptance as a hallowed precept by the profession.[4] More importantly, they believe the emphasis should shift away from a headlong rush to implement the abstract conceptions and definitions of professionalism that have been identified by academic experts and authorities as appropriate content for medical education, and toward a more rigorous continuing discourse regarding the meaning and implications of this movement for learners, teachers, and patients. They further introduce the importance of context in defining and implementing professionalism. In the second piece, Leach addresses the need to find some way to understand professionalism so that it can be applied to individuals and made a part of the process of maturation, or formation, of physicians.[5]

TWO FACES OF PROFESSIONALISM

This dilemma suggests that professionalism may be perceived in different ways by persons operating with different frames of reference. The image of the Roman god Janus, who is portrayed as having two aspects, or faces, each looking in a different direction, suggests itself as a useful metaphor. On the one hand, one face may view professionalism writ large and as a glowing ideal for medicine, calling up different images and different conceptualizations of the profession in society than does the other face, questing after the personal, internalized qualities exemplified in the good physician.

It also suggests that it might be useful to look for ways in which other disciplines or fields have approached such conceptual and operational dilemmas. In this case, I propose that we might do well to borrow an established way of viewing and treating such dilemmas from the field of economics. Hopefully, this will help us create a useful framework for developing theory, as well as more effective ways of designing educational programs and promoting professionalism in medicine.

I refer, of course, to the constructive focus on the qualifiers "micro" and "macro" to distinguish and accommodate different phenomena, different spheres of application, and different levels of abstraction. Such an approach presumably would enable us, then, to identify macroprofessionalism, or professionalism as an ideal, writ large upon the screen of the profession and society. As such, it is often perceived and advanced as an ideological or moral force countering the incursions of commercialization and technology in medicine. On the other hand, microprofessionalism, or professionalism as "formation," to borrow Leach's term, would be seen as applying to a personal developmental process that can be taught or transmitted and in which individuals can participate. Even more to the point, it would enable us to return to the more enlightening process of asking the appropriate questions about professionalism, rather than rushing to implement ill-formed answers and programs that may merely reflect the goals and habits of tradition and establishment.

Macroprofessionalism

To expand further on this concept, macroprofessionalism would be seen as holding on high the more formal values and principles of the profession in society and establishing the standards, rules, and roles that social organizations and institutions play in human interactions. It would also include the expressed ideals, aspirations, and attributions, as well as the societal forms, norms, roles, and structures that have evolved to serve these. This aspect, or face, of professionalism, then, would gaze outward and look more like some of the other important sociomoral constructs that serve to elevate the ideals and aspirations of mankind, such as spirituality, morality, and humanism.

Appropriate questions at this macro level might be aimed at defining the extent and limits of society's contract with medicine and the responsibilities and privileges of achieving and maintaining public trust and confidence, as well as serving to guarantee equality of opportunity, access, and treatment; meeting the needs of both physicians and patients; and securing fairness of costs and rewards and protection from abuse and exploitation. Within this macro concept, then, organizations or institutions would be regarded as operating in a highly professional, socially constructive manner to the extent that they demonstrate or exemplify meritorious attention to the above concerns, conducting themselves in accord with the highest standards of integrity, accountability, and transparency. This, in turn, would presumably result in the rewards of high public esteem, and recognition in the form of increased social support in all its forms. Under certain conditions, the leadership of such organizations might be considered as exemplary, or highly professional, to the extent that their conduct, behavior, and leadership facilitate or are attuned to these same ideals.

In addressing this macro aspect of professionalism, people across a broad range of disciplines and backgrounds invariably tend to fall back on a list of values, attitudes, and behaviors considered as ideal or exemplary in the conduct of human interaction, terms describing the appropriate characteristics and qualities or attributes that persons perceived as being highly professional should be expected to exemplify in thought, intention, and behavior. Various listings of these have appeared in the writings and exhortations of any number of medical authors and organizations, some of which are mentioned previously and appear in figures 8.1 and 8.2.[6]

In an effort to better understand whether and to what degree practicing physicians view these terms as exemplifying professionalism, several years ago some colleagues and I compiled a list of twenty of these terms and descriptors from the literature and asked 187 orthopedists to rate each of them on a scale of one to seven in accord with their personal definition of professionalism. The most highly rated, and therefore presumably most highly regarded, turned out to relate closely to what one would call the work of physicians and included integrity, trustworthiness, responsibility, reliability, duty, and accountability.[7] To our surprise, those qualities and values often spoken of in the literature as most exemplifying professionalism, such as altruism, charity, prudence, temperance, and virtue, were rated lower and ranked at, or near, the bottom of the list. Actually, we probably should not have been surprised to find that, with the exception of integrity, the highly ranked terms largely represent essential, observable work-related behaviors, while the low-ranking ones represent values or personal qualities, which are much more difficult to define and to measure.

Over the past five years, using a slightly expanded list of twenty-five terms, I have continued to collect such information, and I now have data from over five hundred physicians in a number of specialties. The first general observation has been the consistency of the ratings of these terms by practitioners of different ages, backgrounds, and specialties. At first glance, this would appear to be rather reassuring, since it would seem desirable for physicians to see professionalism in the same terms. Indeed, while we had initially speculated

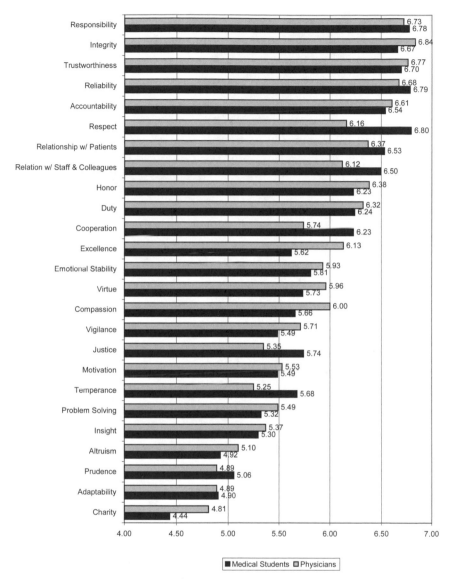

Figure 8.1.   Ratings by Entering Medical Students (N = 105) and Practicing Physicians (N = 498) of How Each Concept Defines Professionalism

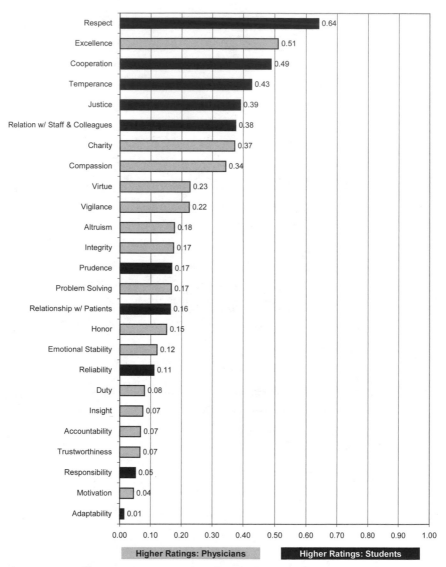

Figure 8.2.   Differences in Ratings of Professionalism Concepts by Entering Medical Students and Practicing Physicians

that there might be some differences based on the nature and demands of their work and the kind of patients and problems encountered, to date we have not found major differences in the ratings or rank order of the attributes by the different specialties. The sole exception has been the slightly higher rankings given by pediatricians to the items dealing with relationships with patients, staff, and colleagues.[8]

In earlier work, I also attempted to make the case for viewing professionalism in a developmental framework, as a dynamic rather than static construct.[9] In an effort to examine this empirically, I asked several colleagues to assist me in obtaining ratings of the same twenty-five terms presented to the older practitioners, from medical students and residents. Again, we were surprised. Although the data are preliminary and limited, rather than observing some sort of progressive, developmental change in the ranking of attributes over the ages and career spans involved, we found that even entering medical students recorded ratings that closely paralleled those of the older practitioners (figure 8.1). At the top of their rankings, both students and practitioners listed the largely work-related attributes of integrity, trustworthiness, responsibility, reliability, and accountability, with virtually no differences in their scores. Similarly, both groups placed the attributes frequently listed as central to the construct of professionalism, such as altruism, charity, prudence, temperance, and justice, at or near the bottom of their rankings, again with little disagreement among them.

Figure 8.2 examines those differences that did emerge between the ratings of the students and the practitioners. Overall, students rated nine of the twenty-five items more highly than did the practitioners. These included (in descending order): respect, cooperation, temperance, justice, relationships with staff and colleagues, prudence, relationships with patients, reliability, and responsibility. The items generally favored by the practitioners included many of the attributes generally ascribed to professionalism in the literature, including charity, compassion, virtue, altruism, integrity, honor, trustworthiness, responsibility, and accountability. In terms of the degree of their differences, seven of the items, nearly all of them the work-related items listed above, differed very slightly (0.08 or less). This supports the overall convergence of thinking by both students and practitioners on these items. On the other hand, there were comparatively large differences of 0.34 or greater on eight items, with respect showing the largest single difference (0.64). Indeed, among these more widely disparate items, the students rated respect, cooperation, temperance, justice, and relationships with staff and colleague more highly than did the practitioners, who gave their higher ratings to excellence, charity, and compassion. Closer examination of the qualities rated more highly by the students suggests that they are ones generally involved in

defining and sustaining human relationships and, therefore, seemingly most
vulnerable to negative or abusive elements in the learning and work environment of medical school and residency.[10] Wear and Kuczewski make this point
in emphasizing the importance of context in the formation of professionalism.[11]

The relative uniformity of perceptions concerning the nature and attributes
of professionalism on the part of established physicians, as well as by entering students, as reported in the previous figures, appears to support the notion
that this aspect, or face, of professionalism is more closely related to a gener-
alizable, or macro, social construct and to certain ideals of the profession than
to a personally achievable competency that can be placed in an individualized, developmental, or maturational framework accessible to educational
programming. It also suggests that macroprofessionalism is fairly well recognized and commonly accepted. As such, it seems to constitute a standard by
which persons performing well in the more highly ranked ways alluded to
previously may be recognized and rewarded as being more professional than
their less exemplary peers. However, nowhere do these findings suggest a
practical or operational way or method for teaching others, especially
younger colleagues, how to attain these qualities, especially since one of the
most frequently recommended methods for imparting professionalism is role
modeling, a method that itself defies precise pedagogical definition.

Microprofessionalism

> "Can you tell me, Socrates—can virtue be taught? Or if not, does it come by
> practice? Or does it come neither by practice nor by teaching, but do people
> get it by nature, or in some other way."[12]

As suggested above, the term "microprofessionalism" would appear to be
more concerned with the day-to-day, face-to-face quality of relationships
with people. It involves such qualities as respect, honesty, integrity, responsibility, trustworthiness, compassion, and cooperation—indeed, many of the
attributes on the list referred to above. However, these qualities are now put
into the context of interpersonal relationships, and that implies and involves
the obligation to comport oneself in those particular ways in our dealings
with one another, including colleagues, staff, and patients. The problem, then,
is, how does one—indeed, can one—learn all there is to know about those
qualities and attributes, and, even more importantly, make them an integral
part of one's behavior and all one does? This is no small task, especially
when most of them are not simply cognitive, but deeply subjective, internalized beliefs and values and engrained habits of living and being.

Obviously, they allude to and require a more limited and individualized or internal developmental process of professional identity formation. Leach frames this aspect, or face, of professionalism in the language of formation, as described by Palmer.[13] The process of formation assumes that every person has access to an "inner teacher," and to the "hidden wholeness" of truth and "inner clarity" to be found or discovered within oneself, which provides an abiding source of guidance and strength in meeting and reflecting on life's deepest issues. The emergence of such inner learning or tacit knowing, however, often involves a response to an outer stimulus of some kind, as demonstrated in Socrates' method of inquiry (maieutics) with the slave Menon quoted above. Another major way of learning and acquiring such desired attributes is by close observation and imitation of advanced masters in the field (role modeling).

Supporting this formative, developmental process, Dreyfus has proposed seven stages, or levels, of progression, or increasing attainment of excellence and mastery, starting with the stage of novice (e.g., an entering medical student), and proceeding up through the levels of advanced beginner (perhaps a senior student), competence (a resident), proficiency (a senior resident or fellow), to expertise (experienced junior faculty), and finally, mastery (senior faculty).[14] Some, hopefully, eventually achieve the final level of "phronesis," or practical wisdom (recognized role models in the field).

These stages appear to be ones that are uniquely appropriate to the micro processes of individual learning, development, and maturation, as summarized in the concept of formation. In the early stages, one learns the language, history, knowledge, and principles of the profession and, particularly, the rules that govern most expected contingencies. In later stages, as problems multiply and become more complex, and simple rules fail, one learns about the exceptions to the rules and what to do when the unexpected occurs. One learns to use intuition and experience to adapt to situations that are novel or unique. Farther along in this process, one observes and models after masters in the field, eventually developing one's own unique style and insight. In the end, one hopes to achieve phronesis, or the practical wisdom to know "exactly which rule to break and exactly how far to break it to accommodate the reality before you."[15] It is important to realize that this process is not smooth or painless. Leaving the certainties of the known and venturing into the complexity and chaos of the unknown is a challenging but essential pathway to mastery and wisdom. Understanding this process of learning and maturation also serves to remind us of what we know about the important social science concepts of socialization and professionalization, which in turn should help us resolve the issue of whether, and how, professionalism can be taught to those entering the profession.

PROFESSIONALISM AS A
DEVELOPMENTAL PROCESS

I have suggested elsewhere that professionalism must recognize the implicit nature of its own developmental processes and structure, as well as its developmental imperative for individuals.[16] Professionalism does not simply spring forth, fully formed, as if from the brow of Zeus. It evolves or comes to fruition, if at all, as something recognized as professionalism at a certain point in time and place only as a result of satisfactory prior and ongoing development and maturation of several other essential components of personality and character. Rather than being achieved simply by doing, or by accomplishing something, it is attained gradually, if at all, as a result of both inner and outer experience, and by a process of action and reflection and formation.[17]

Judith Andre sees this process as essentially a moral endeavor, one involving moral development and the achievement of moral maturity. In turn, this involves "perception, emotion, habitual action, skills in reflection, virtues like courage, patience, and perseverance, and more."[18] These qualities are acquired only gradually and are often accompanied by some personal emotional cost. Hilfiker claims that the experience of failure and its acceptance is an important part of becoming a full self, while Fowler has postulated the necessity of experiencing what he calls the "sacrament of defeat" in achieving true moral maturity.[19] Dreyfus also speaks of the need for an experience of frustration and failure to force one to move beyond the safety and comfort of certainty and rule-bound decision making and face the anxieties of uncertainty.[20] A small example of the often painful process of becoming more professional can be gleaned from the following anecdote. A respected senior physician was once asked by an admiring young resident what made him such a great clinician. He replied, "Good judgment." Queried as to how he had obtained good judgment, the physician answered, "Experience." When further pursued as to how he gained such experience, he responded, "Bad judgment." Becoming truly professional and acquiring wisdom are not for the superficial or impatient.

TOWARD A DEVELOPMENTAL
MODEL OF PROFESSIONALISM

As outlined earlier, I believe that professionalism, seen here as composed of certain values, attitudes, and behaviors, evolves only if based upon, and inclusive of, the prior attainment of an understanding and practice of the values, attitudes, and behaviors consonant with the resolution of the basic existential questions and concerns of three other closely related characterological dimensions, namely, spirituality, morality, and humanism.[21] I have proposed that these important constructs are intimately interrelated in the personal growth and maturation of individuals. I see them as developing in persons sequentially over time, both separately and eventually joined in concert, in a progressive, predictable, interactive, and epigenetic process that closely resembles and is analogous to other developmental phenomena observed in the body and throughout nature. Equally important, I believe that significant deficiencies or interruptions in this process will necessarily result in developmental scars or defects leading to lacunae that, without remediation, will persist into later life and impede full personal achievement of these basic elements of character. Further, as in normal growth and development, there are critical periods for the emergence, engagement, and integration of these guiding constructs, and failure to learn how to deal successfully with the attendant issues and problems at each level or stage will result in future impairment or deficit. Specifically, the model posits that deficit or defect in the critical antecedent elements of spirituality, morality, and/or humanism will inevitably affect the full development of professionalism.

In an earlier work, I presented a visual three-dimensional model of such a progressive, epigenetic, iterative, and developmental process.[22] This model represented the evolving constructs of spirituality, morality, humanism, and professionalism in an ascending sequence from lower left (chronologically and developmentally earlier) to upper right (chronologically and developmentally later) and placed against two defining axes representing the balance or tension between the polar concepts of *internal* versus *external* on the vertical axis, and *self* versus *other* on the horizontal axis (see figure 8.3). In general, there is growth or progress in maturation as individuals shift or expand their orientations from internal to external and from self to other. The model gradually enlarges as it evolves in order to accommodate the continuing and necessary aggregation and integration of learning and experience in each of the individual constructs, as well as in the emerging total body of character and personality. In this sense, the model is holographic, in that any part contains the essential elements, or DNA, of the whole self. Finally, it is expected that these will eventually be manifested in specialty choices that tend to enhance expression of personal and professional interests and talents.

It is extremely important not to interpret the visual and spatial limitations of the two-dimensional representation of the model in figure 8.3 as meaning that each construct is self-limited as to time or space. Although this model

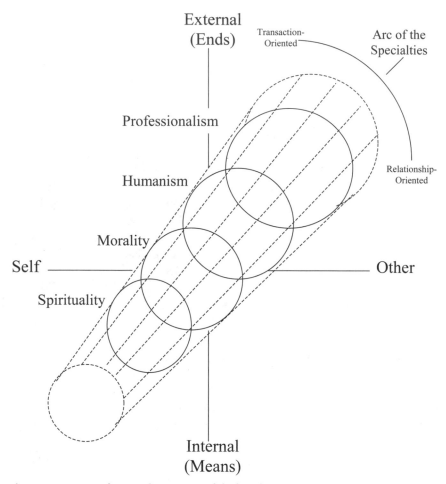

Figure 8.3. Toward a Development Model of Professionalism

posits that these constructs emerge at different developmental and chronological times in the life cycle, they do so in the demonstrated sequence and do not conclude or end at different times. In fact, it is vital that each construct be seen as an active, permanent strand, or essence, however well realized, of the entire being of the person, interacting with, contributing to, and affecting the other constructs. In a life fully lived, spirituality, morality, and humanism do not cease growing but merge into the wholeness of the maturing person. These finally begin to manifest, or take form, as professionalism at the time when the individual enters the flow of his or her life work.

SOME IMPLICATIONS FOR
TEACHING PROFESSIONALISM

The emergent, evolving, and adaptive nature of this conceptual model appears to be consistent with current complexity and chaos theories, as well as with their educational implications. This would suggest that attempting to teach professionalism to entering medical students may be both premature and ineffectual, since it implies and involves issues of professional conduct and relationships that are not in the immediate experience or province of novices or beginners. My experience has been that first- and second-year students are still too new at the game, still at the level of learning facts and rules on one hand, and dealing with the existential questions appropriate to their stage in life on the other, to satisfactorily understand and integrate the issues of professionalism. I believe that the questions entering medical students are asking of themselves and of others are more relevant to the constructs of spirituality (meaning and purpose, being and nonbeing), morality (honesty and dishonesty, ethical and unethical behavior), and humanism (acceptance and rejection, dependence and independence, cooperation and competition) than to those of professionalism. These questions undoubtedly begin to change as students begin their clinical work, but as Feudtner, Christakis, and Christakis and others have shown, many third- and fourth-year medical students are (appropriately) uncomfortable about being called "Doctor," and are expected to be team players and to go along with sometimes questionable decisions made by the clinical team.[23] At this stage, many of their questions concern their responsibilities to and relationships with both their new clinical colleagues and patients. These, I believe, are the early questions relevant to entering professional life and thus to the teaching of professionalism. Teaching, at least in this area, needs to proceed from and be tuned to the issues most relevant and of concern to students at their respective stages of development. As Paul Tillich has said, "The fatal pedagogical error is to throw answers, like stones, at the heads of those who have not yet asked the questions."[24]

The teaching of professionalism to students, then, ideally should emerge from their own questions, as Wear and Kuczewski have suggested.[25] Hopefully, these would be educed in a Socratic (maieutic) manner, in which the students, like the slave Menon, discover their own answers and become aware of their own truths, as they set out on the path to professionalism. This is generally best obtained by engaging them in constructive and instructive discourse, involving current real-life problems and issues, in the presence of mutually reinforcing relationships with respectful fellow learners and teachers, where diversity of viewpoint is encouraged and opinions challenged.

These are precisely the conditions under which it has been shown that students are enabled to make significant gains in moral reasoning.[26] While few learning environments are able to achieve this consistently, true professionalism is more likely to be learned and fostered to the extent that these elements are present. In this regard, I have found that engaging students and practitioners in the discussion of their own results on the professionalism rating scale, described in figures 8.1 and 8.2, has been both stimulating and instructive.

SOME FINAL THOUGHTS

One interesting facet of the literature on professionalism is that, to date, most of the empirical research has highlighted negative, or unprofessional, actions or behaviors rather than positive, professional ones.[27] Much of this reflects the problems around perception and definition addressed earlier in this chapter. It probably also reflects the absorption with the disease, or "deficit," model generally favored by the practice of medicine, which has led researchers in the past to focus more on what is negative, or unprofessional, than on what is properly professional. The assessment of negative and positive qualities has been shown to take place independently of each other.[28] In general, we tend to see the world around us as multidimensional, in that it is possible to see both positive and negative qualities as coexisting in the same individual or situation. Our conceptual view of professionalism may have been lacking in that we have failed to see professional behavior as reflecting both positive and negative dimensions, and as a matter of dynamic tension and choice rather than one of rules and definition. Professionalism, in its final form, then, may be less a competency with known attributes than the capability of actively responding to uncertainty and even chaos with discrimination and judgment.

Ideally, the truly professional physician would aim at using good means or methods to achieve positive outcomes. At the same time, he or she must avoid both bad ends and means. The physician who fails to do either or both of these, then, would generally be considered to be performing in an unprofessional manner. Since these decisions are not always clearly or easily understood, intention becomes an important consideration. A good person is one who strives to do right in all situations. There may be times, however, when he or she may not fully succeed. If he or she recognizes it and makes appropriate repair or restitution, it may be called an error, or mistake, and the person may be forgiven, especially if the intention to strive for the right is clear.[29] The truly unprofessional person, on the other hand, would either fail to comprehend or understand the moral and ethical issues involved (understandable in the case of a beginner or novice) or risk being guilty of excessive hubris by ignoring or defying accepted norms. Bosk labels the latter actions "moral errors" and calls for professional sanction.[30] There may even be times when a positive outcome could conceivably justify the use of negative methods or means, but only if perceived as being undertaken to avoid a more serious wrong. Using this perspective, then, we are required to examine both the ends and the means used by a person, as well as his or her intentionality, in assessing professionalism.

CONCLUSION

In closing, I would like to return to the metaphor of the Roman god Janus, and his two faces. Janus also gave his name to the first month of the year and is known as the god of beginnings. Perhaps we are really just beginning our real study and understanding of what professionalism means in the rapidly changing environment of medical teaching and practice, and how to transmit it to those who follow. Perhaps, too, we have failed to perceive the current thrust and popularity of professionalism for what it really is—a reaction and a response to our antiquated and technologically dominated systems of health care and medical education, and a plea for a medical education consistent with and appropriate to the emerging theories of complexity and of chaos.

NOTES

1. Plato, *Great Dialogues,* eds. E. H. Warmington and P. G. Rouse, trans. W. H. D. Rouse (New York: New American Library, 1936).
2. D. C. Baldwin Jr., unpublished data.
3. L. Carroll, *Through the Looking Glass,* (New York: HarperCollins, 1993), 124.
4. D. Wear and M. G. Kuczewski, "The Professionalism Movement: Can We Pause?" *American Journal of Bioethics* 4 (2004): 1–10.
5. D. C. Leach, "Professionalism: The Formation of Physicians," *American Journal of Bioethics* 4 (2004): 11–12.
6. American Board of Internal Medicine, *Project Professionalism* (Philadelphia: American Board of Internal Medicine, 1994).
7. B. D. Rowley, D. C. Baldwin Jr., R. C. Bay, and R. R. Karpman, "Professionalism and Professional Values in Orthopaedics," *Clinical Orthopaedics and Related Research* 378 (2000): 90–96.
8. Baldwin, unpublished data.
9. D. C. Baldwin Jr. and W. H. Bunch, "Moral Reasoning, Professionalism, and the Teaching of Ethics to Orthopaedic Surgeons," *Clinical Orthopaedics and Related*

Research 378 (2000): 97–103; D. C. Baldwin Jr., "Toward a Theory of Professional Development: Framing Humanism at Core of Good Doctoring and Pedagogy," in *Enhancing the Culture of Medical Education: Conference proceedings*, 6–10 (New York: Arnold P. Gold Foundation, 2003).

10. D. C. Baldwin Jr., S. R. Daugherty, and E. Eckenfels, "Student Perceptions of Mistreatment and Harassment during Medical School: A Survey of Ten Schools," *Western Journal of Medicine* 155 (1991): 140–45; D. C. Baldwin Jr. and S. R. Daugherty, "Do Residents Also Feel 'Abused'? Perceived Mistreatment during Internship," *Academic Medicine* 72 (1997): S51–S53; S. R. Daugherty, D. C. Baldwin Jr., and B. D. Rowley, "Learning, Satisfaction, and Mistreatment during Internship: A National Survey of Working Conditions," *Journal of the American Medical Association* 279 (1998): 1194–99.

11. Wear and Kuczewski, "The Professionalism Movement."

12. Plato, *Great Dialogues.*

13. Leach, "Professionalism"; P. J. Palmer, *To Know as We Are Known: Education as a Spiritual Journey* (San Francisco: HarperSanFrancisco, 1993); P. J. Palmer, *The Courage to Teach* (San Francisco: Jossey-Bass, 1998).

14. H. L. Dreyfus, *On the Internet,* Thinking in Action (London: Routledge, 2001).

15. Attributed to Dr. John Kostis, personal communication with Dr. David Leech, April 24, 2001.

16. Baldwin and Bunch, "Moral Reasoning"; Baldwin, "Toward a Theory of Professional Development."

17. J. Dewey, *Moral Principles in Education* (New York: Philosophical Library, 1954); Palmer, *To Know as We Are Known;* Palmer, *The Courage to Teach.*

18. J. Andre, *Bioethics as Practice* (Chapel Hill: University of North Carolina Press, 2002), 95.

19. D. Hilfiker, *Healing the Wounds* (New York: Penguin, 1987); J. W. Fowler, *Stages of Faith: The Psychology of Human Development and the Quest for Meaning* (San Francisco: Harper & Row, 1981).

20. H. L. Dreyfus, *On the Internet.*

21. Baldwin, "Toward a Theory of Professional Development."

22. Baldwin, "Toward a Theory of Professional Development."

23. C. Feudtner, D. A. Christakis, and N. A. Christakis, "Do Clinical Clerks Suffer Ethical Erosion? Students' Perceptions of Their Ethical Environment and Personal Development," *Academic Medicine* 69 (1994): 670–79.

24. Paul Tillich, quoted at www.thebody.com/atn/406/election.html.

25. Wear and Kuczewski, "The Professionalism Movement."

26. D. J. Self, M. Oliverez, and D. C. Baldwin Jr., "The Amount of Small Group Case Study Discussion Required to Improve Moral Reasoning Skills in Medical Students," *Academic Medicine* 73 (1998): 521–23.

27. D. C. Baldwin Jr. and S. R. Daugherty, "Using Surveys to Assess Professionalism in Individuals and Institutions," in *Measuring Medical Professionalism*, ed. D. Stern, 95–116. (New York: Oxford University Press, 2005).

28. N. Bradburn, *The Structure of Psychological Well-Being* (Chicago: Aldine, 1969).

29. C. L. Bosk, *Forgive and Remember: Managing Medical* Failure (Chicago: University of Chicago Press, 1979).

30. Bosk, *Forgive and Remember.*

List of Contributors

DeWitt C. Baldwin Jr., MD, ScD (hon.), is a scholar-in-residence at the Accreditation Council for Graduate Medical Education in Chicago, Illinois.

Eugene Boisaubin, MD, is professor of medicine and the director of the professionalism curriculum at the University of Texas Medical School at Houston.

Heidi Chang, MPH, is a fourth-year medical student at the Loyola University Chicago Stritch School of Medicine, and is planning a future residency in internal medicine.

Richard Cruess, MD, is professor of surgery and a member of the Centre for Medical Education at McGill University in Montreal, Canada.

Sylvia Cruess, MD, is a professor of medicine and a member of the Centre for Medical Education at McGill University in Montreal, Canada.

Mark A. Farnie, MD, is an associate professor of medicine and pediatrics and is the director of the internal medicine residency training program at the University of Texas Medical School at Houston.

Matthew Fitz, MD, is an assistant professor in internal medicine and pediatrics who directs the internal medicine clerkship at the Loyola University Chicago Stritch School of Medicine, in Maywood, Illinois.

Virginia Greene, BA, is the residency education coordinator for the Department of Internal Medicine at the University of Texas Medical School at Houston.

Frederic W. Hafferty, PhD, is a professor in the Department of Behavioral Sciences at the University of Minnesota Medical School in Duluth, Minnesota.

Mark Kuczewski, PhD, is the Fr. Michael I. English, SJ, Professor of Medical Ethics and the director of the Neiswanger Institute for Bioethics and Health Policy at the Loyola University Chicago Stritch School of Medicine, in Maywood, Illinois.

David C. Leach, M.D., is the executive director of the Accreditation Council for Graduate Medical Education in Chicago, Illinois.

Deirdre C. Lynch, RhD, is a research and evaluation specialist at the Accreditation Council for Graduate Medical Education in Chicago, Illinois.

Aaron J. Michelfelder, MD, is the vice chair of the Department of Family Medicine at the

Loyola University Chicago Stritch School of Medicine, in Maywood, Illinois, where he actively treats patients, educates medical students, and does ethics consultations.

Jing-Bao Nie, BMed, MMed, MA, PhD, is a senior lecturer at the Bioethics Centre at the University of Otago, New Zealand, and author of *Behind Silence: Chinese Voices on Abortion.*

Allison R. Ownby, PhD., MEd, is the assistant director in the Office of Educational Programs and assistant professor in the Department of Pediatrics at the University of Texas Medical School at Houston.

Kayhan Parsi, JD, PhD, is an assistant professor for the Neiswanger Institute for Bioethics and Health Policy, at the Loyola University Chicago Stritch School of Medicine, in Maywood, Illinois.

Myles N. Sheehan, SJ, MD, is senior associate dean for educational programs at the Loyola University Chicago Stritch School of Medicine, in Maywood, Illinois.

Patricia M. Surdyk, PhD, is the executive director for the Institutional Review Committee at the Accreditation Council for Graduate Medical Education in Chicago, Illinois.

Frank Villaume IV, is a fourth-year medical student at the Loyola University Chicago Stritch School of Medicine, in Maywood, Illinois, and is pursuing a career in emergency medicine.

Index